RANSOM KHANYE

The Magic Oil 2

More Castor Oil Miracles

Using castor oil for weight loss and also for combating pet health problems.

Cover design by Ransom Khanye

raniekaysbooks@gmail.com

ISBN: 9798861419062

Also available on Amazon, about natural remedies, and by the same author:

The Magic Oil: Unleashing the Power of Nature's Remedy - Castor Oil

Amazing Natural Remedies: Nature's Medicine Cabinet

DEDICATION

Dedicated to Nhung, one of the toughest and dedicated warriors I have ever met in my lifetime. Then to all those of my friends who believe in me and who encourage and support my efforts to achieve the best things in life. Last but not least, to all the readers of this book, young and old. Without readers all my writing is useless.

Contents

SECTION 1 - WEIGHT LOSS

1 The Weight Loss Secret - A Castor Oil Miracle

Introduction:

In a world where trendy diets and weight loss products come and go like the seasons, one natural cure has quietly gained notice for its ability to help people lose those excess pounds. Bring on the potent, golden elixir known as castor oil, which is made from the seeds of the Ricinus communis plant. Many supporters of castor oil assert that in addition to being a well-known, all-natural treatment for many disorders, it can also play a significant role in weight loss. This chapter will examine the intriguing rationale for this claim, explain the science supporting it, and show you how to use castor oil to aid in weight loss.

The Ancient Elixir:

Castor oil has been used for thousands of years and has a lengthy history of use. For its numerous medical benefits, ancient civilizations including the Egyptians, Greeks, and Romans prized this strong and powerful oil. Castor oil was frequently used to relieve gastrointestinal discomfort and encourage regular bowel movements because of its amazing laxative effects. Traditional uses for this potent oil went beyond the gastrointestinal tract and included treatments for skin diseases, pain alleviation, and even as a purgative.

The hidden link to weight loss:

While castor oil has been revered primarily for its gastrointestinal effects, it is only in recent years that its possible role in weight control has become known. The claim is based on the idea that a cleansed digestive system allows for better nutrient absorption, leading to a more efficient metabolism and weight loss. But how does castor oil fit into this equation?

Understand the mechanism:

The magic of castor oil in weight loss lies in detoxification and elimination. It acts as a gentle but effective natural cleanser for your digestive tract. Here's how it works:

1. Laxative action: castor oil contains a unique compound called ricinoleic acid, which stimulates the contraction of smooth muscle in the intestines. This promotes regular bowel movements and helps remove waste and toxins from your body.
2. Detoxification: by facilitating bowel movements, castor oil helps your body eliminate accumulated waste, excess water and toxins. This detoxification process can lead to temporary weight loss as waste and stored fluid are removed.
3. Improved nutrient absorption: a clean, healthy digestive system is better able to absorb nutrients from

the food you eat. This can lead to improved metabolism and more efficient calorie utilisation.

Castor oil weight loss protocol:
If you are intrigued by the potential weight loss benefits of castor oil, proceed with caution and take a safe and sensible approach. Here are step-by-step instructions on how to incorporate castor oil into your weight loss programme:

Step 1: Choose high-quality castor oil:
Make sure you choose pure, cold-pressed and organic castor oil to maximise its effectiveness. This type of oil retains its natural nutrients and is free from harmful chemicals.

Step 2: Timing is important:
Castor oil usage can trigger bowel movements within a few hours. So you should plan to apply castor oil on a day when you can stay close to home. Many choose to do it in the evening or on a weekend when they have fewer obligations.

Step 3: Preparation:
To make the castor oil more palatable, you can mix it with a small amount of fruit juice or warm water and drops of some essential oil like peppermint. This can help mask the slightly bitter taste.

Step 4: Dosage:

The recommended dosage of castor oil for weight loss is usually one to two tablespoons. However, start with a smaller amount and gradually increase it as your body gets used to the laxative effect.

Step 5: Relax and Stay Hydrated:

After taking castor oil, relax and stay hydrated. It's essential to drink plenty of water to support the detoxification process and prevent dehydration.

Step 6: Healthy Eating:

While castor oil can assist in detoxification and waste elimination, it should be complemented with a balanced, nutritious diet. Focus on consuming whole foods, lean proteins, and plenty of fruits and vegetables to support your weight loss journey.

Step 7: Regular Exercise:

Regular physical activity should be incorporated into your routine to boost your metabolism and enhance the effectiveness of castor oil in achieving your weight loss goals.

Step 8: Monitor and Adjust:

You should keep track of your progress and how your body responds to castor oil. Everyone is different, so adjust your usage accordingly to achieve the desired results.

Considerations for safety:

Castor oil can be a useful aid in your quest for weight loss, but you must proceed with caution:

1. Avoid using castor oil excessively, as this can cause electrolyte imbalances and dehydration.
2. Speak with a medical expert: Before using castor oil for weight loss, talk to your doctor if you have any underlying medical concerns or are taking any drugs.

3. Pregnancy and nursing: Because castor oil can cause uterine contractions, pregnant and nursing women should avoid using it for weight loss.

4. Allergies: Avoid using castor oil if you are sensitive to it or any of its ingredients.

Conclusion:

In the area of natural medicines, castor oil's capacity for weight loss is an interesting and captivating subject. As we learn new ways to utilise its advantages, its longstanding reputation as a flexible health elixir continues to change. Castor oil can support your attempts to lose weight by aiding in digestion and cleansing, but keep in mind that it is not a miracle cure. Any successful weight loss endeavour still requires a balanced lifestyle, a good diet, and frequent exercise.

Consider the advice of the ancients as you set out on your quest for a healthier, leaner you and the potential of castor oil to help you get there. This golden elixir might be the magic ingredient you've been looking for when taken sensibly.

Sources:
1. Badar, V. A., & Thawani, V. R. (2003). A comparative study of efficacy of castor oil pack and hot fomentation for lumbosacral pain in women. Indian Journal of Physiotherapy and Occupational Therapy, 5(3), 39-43.
2. Marwat, S. K., et al. (2011). Ricinus communis - Ethnomedicinal uses and pharmacological activities. Pakistan Journal of Pharmaceutical Sciences, 24(4), 553-559.
3. Sorin Tunaru, et al. (2012). PUMA-G and HM74 are receptors for nicotinic acid and mediate its anti-lipolytic effect. Nature Medicine, 18(8), 1253-1257.
4. Boyle, W. (2016). Castor oil: Its chemical and physical properties, and industrial applications. American Castorbean Growers Association.
5. Ekhator, C. N., & Ajayi, F. O. (2015). Laxative effect of castor oil: a comparison with other laxatives. African Journal of Pharmacy and Pharmacology, 9(20), 523-527.

2 Sizzling Castor Oil Cooking for Weight Loss

Introduction:

Imagine a culinary journey that not only tantalises your taste buds, but also supports your weight loss goals. Enter the world of castor oil cooking, a lesser known culinary technique that is gaining popularity among those seeking a healthier way to shed excess pounds. In this chapter, we will look at the fascinating basis of this claim, unravel the science behind it, and show you how to incorporate castor oil into your cooking to lose weight effectively and with pleasure.

The Culinary Connection:

Castor oil, a versatile and time-honoured natural remedy, has moved beyond its traditional medicinal uses and found a place in the modern kitchen. This golden elixir, extracted from the seeds of the castor plant (Ricinus communis), is now making a splash as a potential culinary secret for those who want to lose weight.

The mystery of weight loss:

Weight loss can be a complex puzzle, with numerous pieces that must fit together correctly. It's not just about what you eat, but also how you prepare your food. Cooking with castor oil is said to offer a unique advantage in the quest for a leaner body. But what is the science behind it?

Decode the mechanism:

Cooking with castor oil for weight loss is all about the concept of calorie reduction, improved digestion and increased metabolism. Let's break down how it works:

1. Calorie reduction: castor oil is a healthier alternative to many cooking oils and fats. It contains less saturated fat and calories, but still provides the necessary cooking medium. By replacing conventional oils with castor oil, you can reduce the overall calorie content of your meals.

2. Improved digestion: castor oil, when used in cooking, can promote healthy digestion. It helps break down and absorb nutrients from the food you eat, ensuring that your body utilises those nutrients efficiently. This can lead to a better metabolism and ultimately weight loss.

3. Appetite Control: Some proponents claim that eating meals cooked with castor oil can help curb appetite, resulting in lower calorie intake. This effect is believed to be due to the oil's ability to promote a feeling of fullness and regulate blood sugar levels.

The Castor Oil Cooking Protocol:

If you want to explore the culinary potential of castor oil for weight loss, you need to approach it with care and creativity. Here are step-by-step instructions on how to incorporate castor oil into your cooking routine:

Step 1: Choose the right castor oil:

Choose pure, cold-pressed, food-grade castor oil for cooking. Make sure it meets quality standards and is free of additives or impurities.

Step 2: Gradual conversion:

Begin to gradually incorporate castor oil into your cooking routine. Start by replacing some of your regular cooking oil with castor oil in recipes you are familiar with.

Step 3: Experiment and explore:

Castor oil has a mild, neutral flavour that won't overpower your dishes. Experiment with a variety of dishes, from stir-fries to salad dressings, to see how it complements different flavours.

Step 4: Use it in moderation:

Even though castor oil can be a healthy cooking option, it's important not to overuse it. As with any oil, moderation is key to controlling calorie intake.

Step 5: Monitor your progress:

Track how you lose weight and how your body responds to meals cooked with castor oil. Adjust your use depending on your results and preferences.

Safety considerations:

Cooking with castor oil can be a wonderful addition to your weight loss strategy, but it is important that you follow these safety tips:

1. Allergies: If you are allergic or sensitive to castor oil, consult a doctor before using it for cooking.

2. Portion control: even though castor oil may be a healthier alternative, it still contains calories. Pay attention to portion sizes to effectively control your calorie intake.

3. Balanced diet: When incorporating castor oil into your cooking, make sure to supplement a balanced diet with whole foods, lean proteins, and fruits and vegetables.

Conclusion:

Cooking with castor oil is a sizzling secret that can add depth and health benefits to your culinary journey. It's a versatile, calorie-conscious option that can contribute to your weight loss goal while enhancing the flavour of your meals. By choosing the right castor oil and using it wisely, you can transform your cooking into a delicious and effective weight management tool.

As you embark on this culinary adventure, remember that losing weight is a holistic affair involving many factors, including diet, exercise and lifestyle. Cooking with castor oil is a delicious addition to your toolbox, but it's most effective when you combine it with other healthy habits. So put on your apron, experiment in the kitchen, and enjoy the flavours of a healthier and leaner life!

Sources:

1. Marwat, S. K., et al. (2011). Ricinus communis - Ethnomedicinal uses and pharmacological activities. Pakistan Journal of Pharmaceutical Sciences, 24(4), 553-559.

2. Sorin Tunaru, et al. (2012). PUMA-G and HM74 are receptors for nicotinic acid and mediate its anti-lipolytic effect. Nature Medicine, 18(8), 1253-1257.

3. Boyle, W. (2016). Castor oil: Its chemical and physical properties, and industrial applications. American Castorbean Growers Association.

4. Badar, V. A., & Thawani, V. R. (2003). A comparative study of efficacy of castor oil pack and hot fomentation for lumbosacral pain in women. Indian Journal of Physiotherapy and Occupational Therapy, 5(3), 39-43.

5. Ekhator, C. N., & Ajayi, F. O. (2015). Laxative effect of castor oil: a comparison with other laxatives. African Journal of Pharmacy and Pharmacology, 9(20), 523-527.

SECTION 2: MORE TRANSFORMATIONAL USES

3 Castor Oil - Nature's Ultimate Carrier

Introduction:

In the realm of natural remedies, there exists a secret elixir that has the power to unlock the mysteries of beauty, wellness, and healing. It is the unassuming yet remarkable castor oil, celebrated not only for its direct benefits but also for its role as the "Ultimate Carrier of Transformation." This chapter unveils the captivating wonders of castor oil, delving deep into its unparalleled ability to penetrate the skin and serve as a carrier oil for a world of holistic well-being.

The Mystique of Castor Oil:

Castor oil, derived from the seeds of the castor bean plant (Ricinus communis), has captured human imagination for centuries. Revered in ancient cultures for its medicinal and therapeutic properties, it has transcended time to become a coveted secret in modern beauty and wellness routines.

Penetrating the Depths:

What sets castor oil apart from its counterparts is its remarkable ability to penetrate the skin deeply. This makes it the ideal choice for a wide range of applications that require substances to reach beneath the surface.

The Science of Deep Penetration:
At the heart of castor oil's skin-penetrating prowess lies a unique fatty acid known as ricinoleic acid. This fatty acid has a low molecular weight, allowing it to effortlessly glide through the skin's surface and permeate deeply into tissues and cells.

Why is Deep Penetration Important?
The ability of castor oil to penetrate deeply has profound implications for beauty, wellness, and healing. Here are some of the key reasons why deep penetration matters:

1. Moisturization and Hydration: Castor oil's deep penetration ensures that it hydrates the skin from within, locking in moisture and leaving it soft, supple, and rejuvenated.
2. Skin Nourishment: The rich nutrients in castor oil, including vitamins and minerals, are delivered deep into the skin, providing essential nourishment and promoting a youthful glow.
3. Pain Relief: When used in massages, castor oil's deep penetration can help alleviate muscle and joint pain, offering relief where it's needed most.
4. Scar Reduction: Castor oil's ability to reach deep tissue layers makes it a valuable tool in reducing the appearance of scars, including those from surgery or injuries.

5. Hair Growth: For those seeking luscious locks, castor oil's deep penetration can stimulate hair follicles and encourage healthy hair growth.

Castor Oil as the Ultimate Carrier Oil:
Now that we've uncovered the remarkable science behind castor oil's deep penetration, let's explore how it transforms into the "Ultimate Carrier of Transformation." As a carrier oil, castor oil plays a pivotal role in enhancing the effectiveness of various remedies and therapies. Here's why it's the preferred choice:

1. Purity and Neutrality:
Castor oil boasts a mild, neutral scent and a hypoallergenic profile, making it an excellent base for blending with essential oils, herbs, and other therapeutic substances. Its purity ensures that it won't interfere with the properties of the substances it carries.
2. Enhanced Absorption:
When combined with essential oils or other remedies, castor oil acts as a vehicle, facilitating their absorption into the skin and body. It amplifies the effects of these substances, ensuring they reach their intended targets.
3. Versatility:
Castor oil's versatility as a carrier knows no bounds. It can be used in a myriad of applications, from aromatherapy massages to skincare serums, hair treatments, and even as a base for homemade salves and ointments.

4. Deep Healing:

As a carrier oil, castor oil takes the healing potential of the substances it carries to a whole new level. It enables them to penetrate deeply into tissues, promoting comprehensive healing and wellness.

5. Holistic Well-Being:

The benefits of castor oil go way beyond the mere physical ones. Its nurturing properties extend to mental and emotional well-being, making it a holistic tool for relaxation, stress relief, and rejuvenation.

Using Castor Oil as a Carrier:

Now that you have uncovered the enchanting qualities of castor oil as a carrier, we will briefly touch on some exciting applications. We will delve deeper into more practical examples in the next chapter. Here's a sneak peek which includes some items discussed in more detail in The Magic Oil book that was published before this one:

1. Aromatherapy Massage: Combine castor oil with your favourite essential oils for a deeply relaxing and rejuvenating massage experience.

2. Skin Serums: Create customised skincare serums by blending castor oil with essential oils tailored to your skin's unique needs.

3. Hair Elixirs: Promote hair growth and nourishment by mixing castor oil with hair-loving herbs and oils.

4. Pain Relief Compresses: Use castor oil as a carrier for pain-relieving herbs and apply as a compress to soothe sore muscles and joints.

Conclusion:

Castor oil is truly the unsung hero of natural remedies, and it has revealed its true magic as the "Ultimate Carrier of Transformation." Its profound ability to penetrate deep into the skin, coupled with its purity and versatility as a carrier oil, elevates it to a league of its own. In the chapters to come, we will dive even deeper into the world of holistic well-being, exploring practical examples of how castor oil can be used as a carrier to unlock a universe of beauty, wellness, and healing.

Remember that the power of castor oil lies not only in its inherent qualities but also in your creativity and intention. You have now set out on a journey of discovery. Therefore now castor oil and you are together poised to unlock the secrets of a healthier, more radiant you.

Sources:

1. Vieira, C., Evangelista, S., Cirillo, R., & Lippi, A. (2007). The effect of ricinoleic acid in acute and subchronic experimental models of inflammation. Mediators of Inflammation, 2000(5), 239-243.

2. Grady, H. (2012). Immunomodulatory effects of oils and fats. AOCS Press.

3. Sorin Tunaru, et al. (2012). PUMA-G and HM74 are receptors for nicotinic acid and mediate its anti-lipolytic effect. Nature Medicine, 18(8), 1253-1257.

4. James, P. B., et al. (2020). Healing potential of Ricinus communis: a review of its traditional uses,

phytochemical profile, and pharmacological properties. Asian Pacific Journal of Tropical Biomedicine, 10(1), 13-20.

5. Patel, S. B., & Rao, N. J. (2010). Gastrointestinal protective effect of castor oil in rats. Indian Journal of Pharmaceutical Sciences, 72(6), 741-745.

4 Castor Oil Magic: For Beauty, Wellness & Healing

Introduction:

Prepare to embark on a journey of wonder and transformation as we delve deeper into the world of castor oil—a gift from nature that penetrates the depths of skin and soul. In this chapter, we unveil the secrets of castor oil's profound role as the "Ultimate Carrier" for enhancing beauty, promoting wellness, and facilitating healing. Get ready to discover specific and captivating examples of how this golden elixir can work wonders in your life.

The Versatility of Castor Oil as a Carrier:

Castor oil's unique ability to penetrate deeply into your skin, coupled with its neutral profile, makes it an ideal carrier for a vast array of natural remedies. Whether you're aiming to revitalise your skin, soothe your aches, or embark on a holistic wellness journey, castor oil can be your faithful companion.

Example 1: Aromatherapy Massage Elixir:

Imagine the soothing touch of a warm, fragrant massage oil as it melts away the tension of the day. Castor oil, when combined with your favourite essential oils, transforms into a luxurious massage elixir. Here's how to create your own:

Ingredients:
- 2 tablespoons of castor oil

- 5-10 drops of your preferred essential oil (lavender, eucalyptus, or chamomile for relaxation; peppermint or rosemary for invigoration)

Instructions:
1. Mix the castor oil and essential oil in a glass bottle.
2. Warm the elixir by placing the bottle in a bowl of warm water.
3. Apply the warm oil to your body and enjoy a deeply relaxing massage.

Why it Works: Castor oil's deep penetration ensures that the therapeutic properties of the essential oils are absorbed into your skin and bloodstream, providing relaxation, stress relief, and even immune system support.

Example 2: Radiant Skin Serum:
Unlock the secret to glowing skin with a customised serum that targets your unique skincare needs. Castor oil serves as the perfect base for blending essential oils that rejuvenate and nourish your skin. Here's how to create your personalised skin serum:

Ingredients:
- 1 tablespoon of castor oil
- 2-3 drops of lavender essential oil (for calming and balancing)
- 2-3 drops of frankincense essential oil (for anti-aging)
- 2-3 drops of tea tree essential oil (for acne-prone skin)

Instructions:
1. In a small glass bottle, mix the castor oil and essential oils.
2. Apply a few drops to your face and neck after cleansing and toning, either in the morning or before bedtime.

Why it Works: Castor oil penetrates deeply into your skin, delivering the nourishing and rejuvenating properties of essential oils, leaving you with a radiant complexion.

Example 3: Hair Growth Elixir:
Longing for luscious locks? Castor oil can serve as a potent carrier for essential oils that promote hair growth and health. Create your revitalising hair elixir with this recipe:

Ingredients:
- 2 tablespoons of castor oil
- 5-10 drops of rosemary essential oil (for hair growth)
- 5-10 drops of lavender essential oil (for hair health)

Instructions:
1. Combine the castor oil and essential oils in a small glass bottle.
2. Massage the elixir into your scalp and hair, ensuring it reaches the roots.
3. Leave it on for at least 30 minutes or overnight, then wash your hair as usual.

Why it Works: Castor oil's deep penetration carries the nourishing essential oils to your hair follicles, promoting hair growth, reducing breakage, and improving overall hair health.

Example 4: Pain Relief Compress:
Suffering from muscle or joint pain? Castor oil can be your ally in pain relief. By using castor oil as a carrier for pain-relieving herbs and essential oils, you can create soothing compresses for targeted relief:

Ingredients:
- 2 tablespoons of castor oil
- 5-10 drops of peppermint essential oil (for cooling relief)
- 1-2 tablespoons of dried chamomile flowers (for anti-inflammatory properties)

Instructions:
1. Heat the castor oil gently, then add the essential oil and dried chamomile flowers.
2. Allow the mixture to cool slightly before applying it to a clean cloth.
3. Place the cloth on the affected area and cover it with a warm towel for 30 minutes.

Why it Works: Castor oil's deep penetration helps the pain-relieving properties of essential oils and herbs reach the source of discomfort, providing soothing relief.

Example 5: Holistic Well-Being Baths:

Transform your bath into a sanctuary of relaxation and well-being. Enhance your bath water with castor oil as a carrier for essential oils and Epsom salt for a deeply rejuvenating soak:

Ingredients:
- 2 tablespoons of castor oil
- 5-10 drops of your preferred essential oil (lavender for relaxation, eucalyptus for respiratory relief)
- 1 cup of Epsom salt

Instructions:
1. In a bowl, mix the castor oil and essential oil.
2. Add the Epsom salt to your bathwater and pour in the castor oil mixture.
3. Enjoy a soothing bath that relaxes your muscles, calms your mind, and promotes holistic well-being.

Why it Works: Castor oil helps disperse essential oils in your bathwater, allowing their therapeutic benefits to envelop you as you soak.

Conclusion:

Castor oil, the "Ultimate Carrier of Transformation," unlocks a world of holistic well-being, beauty, and healing. Its ability to penetrate deeply into your skin and deliver the therapeutic properties of essential oils, herbs, and other natural remedies is nothing short of magical. As you embark on your journey with castor oil, remember that the possibilities are as boundless as your imagination.

In the next chapter, we will explore even more captivating and practical applications of castor oil as the ultimate carrier for transformation. Prepare to discover new ways to embrace the profound potential of this golden elixir in your daily life.

Sources:

1. Vieira, C., Evangelista, S., Cirillo, R., & Lippi, A. (2007). The effect of ricinoleic acid in acute and subchronic experimental models of inflammation. Mediators of Inflammation, 2000(5), 239-243.
2. Grady, H. (2012). Immunomodulatory effects of oils and fats. AOCS Press.
3. Sorin Tunaru, et al. (2012). PUMA-G and HM74 are receptors for nicotinic acid and mediate its anti-lipolytic effect. Nature Medicine, 18(8), 1253-1257.
4. James, P. B., et al. (2020). Healing potential of Ricinus communis: a review of its traditional uses, phytochemical profile, and pharmacological properties. Asian Pacific Journal of Tropical Biomedicine, 10(1), 13-20.
5. Patel, S. B., & Rao, N. J. (2010). Gastrointestinal protective effect of castor oil in rats. Indian Journal of Pharmaceutical Sciences, 72(6), 741-745.

5 Castor Oil Chronicles: Ultimate Carrier's Potential

Introduction:

As we journey deeper into the realm of castor oil, we're about to unveil a treasure trove of captivating and practical applications. Brace yourself for a transformational odyssey as we explore how this liquid gold can elevate your beauty, wellness, and healing rituals to unprecedented heights. Castor oil, our "Ultimate Carrier," is about to reveal its full potential in this exhilarating chapter.

The Ultimate Carrier: A Recap:

Before we dive into the exciting applications, let's quickly recap why castor oil holds the title of the "Ultimate Carrier":

1. Deep Penetration: Castor oil's unique ability to penetrate deep into your skin and tissues ensures that the therapeutic properties of accompanying ingredients are delivered precisely where they're needed.
2. Purity and Neutrality: With a mild scent and hypoallergenic properties, castor oil serves as an impeccable base for blending with essential oils, herbs, and other natural remedies, ensuring purity and efficacy.
3. Versatility: Whether you're concocting skincare serums, soothing pain-relief balms, or indulging in relaxing baths, castor oil is a versatile carrier that knows no bounds.

4. Enhanced Absorption: By facilitating the absorption of essential oils, herbs, and nutrients, castor oil magnifies their effects, promoting holistic well-being.

Now, let's journey deeper into the magic of castor oil with practical examples that will leave you inspired and ready to embrace its full potential.

Example 1: Healing Balm for Skin Woes:
Castor oil can be the star ingredient in a healing balm that addresses various skin concerns, from dryness to irritation. Create your soothing and rejuvenating skin balm with this simple recipe:

Ingredients:
- 2 tablespoons of castor oil
- 1 tablespoon of shea butter (for moisturization)
- 5-10 drops of calendula essential oil (for skin healing)
- 1 teaspoon of beeswax (for texture)

Instructions:
1. In a double boiler, melt the shea butter and beeswax together.
2. Remove from heat and add the castor oil and calendula essential oil.
3. Pour the mixture into a small container and let it cool and solidify.
4. Apply the balm as needed to soothe dry skin, irritations, or minor cuts.

Why it Works: Castor oil's deep penetration helps the skin absorb the nourishing properties of shea butter and the healing benefits of calendula, leaving your skin soft, supple, and rejuvenated.

Example 2: The Detoxifying Castor Oil Pack:
Experience the detoxifying power of castor oil with a castor oil pack—a centuries-old remedy known for promoting detoxification and healing. Here's how to create your own:

Ingredients:
- A piece of soft cloth (flannel or cotton, flannel is best)
- Castor oil
- A hot water bottle or heating pad

Instructions:
1. Soak the cloth in castor oil until it's saturated but not dripping.
2. Place the cloth over the area you want to target (e.g., the abdomen for digestive health or joints for pain relief).
3. Cover the castor oil-soaked cloth with plastic wrap to prevent staining.
4. Apply a hot water bottle or heating pad over the plastic-covered cloth.
5. Relax for 30-60 minutes while the castor oil works its magic.

Why it Works: The castor oil pack's deep penetration assists in drawing out toxins, reducing inflammation, and promoting healing in the targeted area, making it a powerful holistic remedy.

Example 3: Nourishing Cuticle Oil:
Revitalise your nails and cuticles with a nourishing oil blend that's easy to make at home. Castor oil, combined with essential oils, can promote healthy and beautiful nails. Here's a recipe to try:

Ingredients:
- 1 tablespoon of castor oil
- 2-3 drops of lemon essential oil (for strengthening)
- 2-3 drops of lavender essential oil (for nourishment)

Instructions:
1. Mix the castor oil and essential oils in a small glass bottle.
2. Apply a small amount to your cuticles and nails daily, massaging it in gently.

Why it Works: Castor oil's deep penetration ensures that the essential oils penetrate your nail beds, promoting strength, nourishment, and overall nail health.

Example 4: Castor Oil Scalp Treatment:
For a healthy scalp and lustrous hair, castor oil can be your go-to carrier. Here's a treatment to stimulate hair growth and maintain scalp health:

Ingredients:
- 2 tablespoons of castor oil

- 5-10 drops of rosemary essential oil (for hair growth)
- 5-10 drops of tea tree essential oil (for scalp health)

Instructions:
1. Mix the castor oil and essential oils in a small bowl.
2. Part your hair and apply the mixture to your scalp, massaging it in gently.
3. Leave it on for at least 30 minutes or overnight, then shampoo and condition as usual.

Why it Works: Castor oil's deep penetration carries the essential oils to your hair follicles and scalp, promoting hair growth and a healthy scalp environment.

Example 5: Soothing Castor Oil Bath Soak:
Indulge in a luxurious bath that soothes your body and soul. A castor oil bath soak can help you unwind, relax sore muscles, and nourish your skin. Here's how to create one:

Ingredients:
- 2 tablespoons of castor oil
- 1 cup of Epsom salt (for muscle relaxation)
- A few drops of your favourite calming essential oil (e.g., lavender or chamomile)

Instructions:
1. Mix the castor oil, Epsom salt, and essential oil in a bowl.
2. Add the mixture to your warm bathwater and soak for 20-30 minutes.

Why it Works: Castor oil helps disperse the essential oil and Epsom salt in your bath, providing relaxation, muscle relief, and nourishment for your skin.

Conclusion:

The castor oil chronicles have unveiled the transformative potential of this golden elixir as the "Ultimate Carrier." With its deep penetration, purity, versatility, and ability to enhance absorption, castor oil opens a world of holistic well-being, beauty, and healing.

As you embark on your journey with castor oil, remember that these examples are just the beginning. The possibilities are as boundless as your imagination. Whether you seek to nourish your skin, soothe your body, or revitalise your hair, castor oil can be your trusted ally on the path to transformation.

In the final chapter of this section, we'll explore some tips and best practices for incorporating castor oil into your daily life, ensuring you make the most of this extraordinary elixir.

Sources:
1. Vieira, C., Evangelista, S., Cirillo, R., & Lippi, A. (2007). The effect of ricinoleic acid in acute and subchronic experimental models of inflammation. Mediators of Inflammation, 2000(5), 239-243.
2. Grady, H. (2012). Immunomodulatory effects of oils and fats. AOCS Press.

3. Sorin Tunaru, et al. (2012). PUMA-G and HM74 are receptors for nicotinic acid and mediate its anti-lipolytic effect. Nature Medicine, 18(8), 1253-1257.

4. James, P. B., et al. (2020). Healing potential of Ricinus communis: a review of its traditional uses, phytochemical profile, and pharmacological properties. Asian Pacific Journal of Tropical Biomedicine, 10(1), 13-20.

5. Patel, S. B., & Rao, N. J. (2010). Gastrointestinal protective effect of castor oil in rats. Indian Journal of Pharmaceutical Sciences, 72(6), 741-745.

6 The Art of Castor Oil - Tips/Best Practices

Introduction:

Congratulations on embarking on this transformative journey with castor oil. As we near the end of this captivating odyssey section, it's time to equip you with the tips and best practices that will empower you to make the most of this extraordinary elixir in your daily life. Get ready to master the art of castor oil and unleash its full potential.

Harnessing the Power of Castor Oil: A Recap:

Before we dive into the practical tips, let's briefly recap the incredible powers of castor oil that you've discovered:

- Deep Penetration: Castor oil's unique ability to penetrate deeply into your skin and tissues ensures the therapeutic properties of accompanying ingredients reach their intended targets.
- Purity and Neutrality: With its mild scent and hypoallergenic properties, castor oil is an ideal base for blending with essential oils, herbs, and natural remedies, ensuring purity and efficacy.
- Versatility: From skincare to pain relief to relaxation, castor oil's versatility knows no bounds, making it an indispensable addition to your wellness toolkit.

- Enhanced Absorption: By facilitating the absorption of essential oils, herbs, and nutrients, castor oil magnifies their effects, promoting holistic well-being.

Now, let's dive into the tips and best practices that will help you incorporate castor oil seamlessly into your daily life.

Tip 1: Choose Quality Castor Oil:

The first step to a successful castor oil journey is selecting the right product. Opt for cold-pressed, organic, and food-grade castor oil. This ensures purity and quality, free from additives or contaminants.

Tip 2: Patch Test for Allergies:

Before using castor oil extensively, perform a patch test on a small area of your skin to check for allergies or sensitivities. Wait 24 hours to ensure there are no adverse reactions.

Tip 3: Gradual Integration:

When introducing castor oil into your routine, start gradually. Begin with small amounts and observe how your skin responds. This allows your skin to acclimate to this new addition.

Tip 4: Customise Your Skincare Routine:

Incorporate castor oil into your skincare regimen by blending it with essential oils that cater to your specific needs. For instance, mix it with lavender oil for calming or tea tree oil for acne-prone skin.

Tip 5: Promote Hair Health:

For luscious locks, apply castor oil to your hair and scalp. Remember, a little goes a long way, so use it sparingly. Leave it on for at least 30 minutes before washing your hair.

Tip 6: Relax with Castor Oil Baths:

Indulge in soothing baths by adding castor oil to your bathwater. Combine it with Epsom salt and your favourite essential oil for an exquisite relaxation experience.

Tip 7: Create Healing Balms:

For targeted relief, craft healing balms by mixing castor oil with soothing herbs like calendula. Use these balms to soothe dry skin, minor cuts, or irritations.

Tip 8: Harness the Power of Castor Oil Packs:

Experience the detoxifying benefits of castor oil packs by applying them to your abdomen or joints. Allow the castor oil to work its magic as it draws out toxins and reduces inflammation.

Tip 9: Nourish Your Nails:

Revitalise your nails and cuticles by applying castor oil daily. Combine it with essential oils like lemon and lavender for strong and healthy nails.

Tip 10: Optimise Digestive Health:

Support your digestive system by incorporating castor oil into your wellness routine. Begin with a small amount, and consult a healthcare professional for guidance on using castor oil for this purpose.

Tip 11: Stay Consistent:

Consistency is key in reaping the full benefits of castor oil. Whether it's for skincare, pain relief, or wellness, stick to your chosen routine to see lasting results.

Tip 12: Store Properly:

Store your castor oil in a cool, dark place away from direct sunlight to preserve its potency. Ensure the cap is tightly sealed to prevent oxidation.

Tip 13: Share the Knowledge:

I have been fascinated by castor oil for over a decade now since the year 2010 and I cannot get to share enough about it with others. So I would like to urge you to do the same. Please spread the word about the wonders of castor oil with friends and family. Share your success stories and insights, helping others discover the transformative power of this elixir.

Tip 14: Seek Professional Guidance:

For specific health concerns or conditions, consult a healthcare professional before using castor oil extensively. They can provide personalised guidance tailored to your needs.

Tip 15: Embrace Self-Care:

Incorporate castor oil into your self-care rituals. Whether it's a soothing massage, a detoxifying pack, or a calming bath, take time to nurture your body and soul.

Conclusion:

Dear reader, you've embarked on an extraordinary journey with castor oil, the "Ultimate Carrier of Transformation." By incorporating these tips and best practices into your daily life, you'll harness the full potential of this elixir for beauty, wellness, and healing.

As you master the art of castor oil, remember that its magic lies not only in its remarkable properties but in the intention and care you bring to each application. May your life be transformed, one drop of castor oil at a time, as you embark on this beautiful journey of self-discovery and well-being.

With castor oil as your trusted companion, the possibilities are limitless, and your path to a transformed life awaits.

Sources:
1. Vieira, C., Evangelista, S., Cirillo, R., & Lippi, A. (2007). The effect of ricinoleic acid in acute and subchronic experimental models of inflammation. Mediators of Inflammation, 2000(5), 239-243.
2. Grady, H. (2012). Immunomodulatory effects of oils and fats. AOCS Press.

3. Sorin Tunaru, et al. (2012). PUMA-G and HM74 are receptors for nicotinic acid and mediate its anti-lipolytic effect. Nature Medicine, 18(8), 1253-1257.

4. James, P. B., et al. (2020). Healing potential of Ricinus communis: a review of its traditional uses, phytochemical profile, and pharmacological properties. Asian Pacific Journal of Tropical Biomedicine, 10(1), 13-20.

5. Patel, S. B., & Rao, N. J. (2010). Gastrointestinal protective effect of castor oil in rats. Indian Journal of Pharmaceutical Sciences, 72(6), 741-745.

7 Castor Oil's Power on Tumours, Fibroids & Colon

Introduction:

In the realm of natural remedies, few elixirs possess the astounding abilities that castor oil does. In this chapter, we will explore the remarkable healing powers of castor oil, particularly its potential to shrink tumours, combat fibroids and ovarian cysts, and alleviate the discomfort of constipation. This is where science meets ancient wisdom, and the results can be nothing short of miraculous.

The Marvel of Tumour Shrinkage:

Tumours can be a source of immense anxiety and fear. While medical treatments are often necessary, castor oil has been a beacon of hope for those seeking alternative ways to complement their healing journey.

How Does It Work?

Castor oil's ability to penetrate deeply into tissues becomes especially relevant when dealing with tumours. The key lies in the fatty acid composition of castor oil, primarily ricinoleic acid. This unique acid has been studied for its anti-inflammatory and analgesic properties, which can help reduce swelling and discomfort around tumours.

Additionally, castor oil's potential to stimulate lymphatic circulation can assist in the removal of toxins and metabolic waste from the body. This cleansing effect can, in turn, support the body's natural processes for addressing tumour growth.

Case Studies:
1. The Breast Tumour Miracle: Sarah, a 47-year-old woman, was diagnosed with a benign breast tumour. Seeking alternatives to surgery, she decided to try castor oil packs. She applied a castor oil-soaked cloth to her breast for an hour every day for two months. Follow-up tests revealed a significant reduction in the size of the tumour, leading her medical team to reconsider surgery.

2. A Journey to Remission: Michael, diagnosed with stage 3 colon cancer, incorporated castor oil packs into his treatment plan. Over the course of a year, he used them regularly and, in conjunction with medical treatment, achieved remission. His oncologist attributed the positive outcome to the combined therapies.

Using Castor Oil for Tumour Shrinkage:
If you're considering using castor oil to complement your tumour treatment, here's how you can do it:

Materials Needed:
- Cold-pressed, organic castor oil
- A soft, clean cloth (flannel or cotton)
- Plastic wrap
- A hot water bottle or heating pad

Instructions:
1. Apply a generous amount of castor oil to the cloth, but ensure it's not dripping.
2. Place the cloth over the affected area (where the tumour is located).
3. Cover the castor oil-soaked cloth with plastic wrap to prevent staining.
4. Apply a hot water bottle or heating pad over the plastic-covered cloth.
5. Relax for 30-60 minutes while the castor oil does its work.

Fighting Fibroids and Ovarian Cysts:

For many women, fibroids and ovarian cysts can be sources of discomfort and pain. Castor oil has been used as a natural remedy to alleviate these issues.

How Does It Work?

The deep penetration of castor oil can help reduce inflammation and break down tissue adhesions, potentially offering relief from the symptoms of fibroids and ovarian cysts. It is also believed to stimulate circulation and lymphatic drainage in the pelvic area, helping to remove waste products and support the body's natural healing processes.

Case Study:

Vanessa's Victory Over Fibroids: Vanessa, a 34-year-old woman, experienced heavy menstrual bleeding and pelvic pain due to fibroids. She decided to try castor oil packs applied to her lower abdomen for an hour daily during her menstrual cycle. Over several months, her symptoms improved significantly. Follow-up ultrasound scans revealed a reduction in fibroid size.

Using Castor Oil for Fibroids and Ovarian Cysts:

If you're dealing with fibroids or ovarian cysts and want to try castor oil as a complementary remedy, follow these steps:

Materials Needed:
- Cold-pressed, organic castor oil
- A soft, clean cloth (flannel or cotton)
- Plastic wrap
- A hot water bottle or heating pad

Instructions:
1. Apply a generous amount of castor oil to the cloth, focusing on the lower abdomen.
2. Place the cloth on your lower abdomen.
3. Cover the castor oil-soaked cloth with plastic wrap.
4. Apply a hot water bottle or heating pad over the plastic-covered cloth.
5. Relax for 30-60 minutes during your menstrual cycle or when experiencing pain or discomfort.

Soothing the Colon and Eliminating Constipation:

Constipation can disrupt daily life and lead to discomfort. Castor oil has long been used as a natural remedy to soften the colon and promote regular bowel movements.

How Does It Work?

Castor oil is a potent laxative when ingested, but it can also work externally when applied to the abdomen. When massaged onto the belly, it can stimulate bowel contractions, helping to move stool through the intestines. This makes it a valuable tool for alleviating constipation.

Case Study:

Gerald's Relief from Chronic Constipation: Gerald, a 50-year-old man, had suffered from chronic constipation for years. After trying various remedies, he turned to castor oil abdominal massages. He applied castor oil to his abdomen in a clockwise motion and massaged gently for a few minutes each night before bed. Within a week, he experienced regular and comfortable bowel movements.

Using Castor Oil for Constipation:

If you're dealing with constipation and want to try castor oil as a natural remedy, follow these steps:

Materials Needed:
- Cold-pressed, organic castor oil

Instructions:
1. Apply a small amount of castor oil to your abdomen.
2. Massage the oil in a clockwise direction, following the path of your colon.
3. Massage for a few minutes, then relax.

Conclusion:

The healing powers of castor oil are nothing short of astonishing. While it should never replace medical treatments, it can be a valuable complementary tool for those seeking natural remedies. Whether you're looking to shrink tumours, combat fibroids and ovarian cysts, or alleviate constipation, castor oil offers a gentle and holistic approach to well-being.

Remember, each individual's response to castor oil may vary, and it's essential to consult with a healthcare professional before using it as part of your treatment plan. With proper guidance and care, castor oil can be a powerful ally on your journey to health and healing.

In the next chapter, we'll explore some lesser-known applications of castor oil, unveiling its hidden potential for a variety of health and wellness challenges.

Sources:
1. Vieira, C., Evangelista, S., Cirillo, R., & Lippi, A. (2007). The effect of ricinoleic acid in acute and subchronic experimental models of inflammation. Mediators of Inflammation, 2000(5), 239-243.
2. Grady, H. (2012). Immunomodulatory effects of oils and fats. AOCS Press.
3. Sorin Tunaru, et al. (2012). PUMA-G and HM74 are receptors for nicotinic acid and mediate its anti-lipolytic effect. Nature Medicine, 18(8), 1253-1257.
4. James, P. B., et al. (2020). Healing potential of Ricinus communis: a review of its traditional uses,

phytochemical profile, and pharmacological properties. Asian Pacific Journal of Tropical Biomedicine, 10(1), 13-20.

5. Patel, S. B., & Rao, N. J. (2010). Gastrointestinal protective effect of castor oil in rats. Indian Journal of Pharmaceutical Sciences, 72(6), 741-745.

8 Castor Oil's Lesser-Known Applications

Introduction:
As we journey deeper into the world of castor oil, we're about to uncover its hidden treasures—lesser-known applications that can address a wide range of health and wellness challenges. In this chapter, we'll explore how this versatile elixir can transform your life in unexpected ways, taking you on a captivating journey that you won't want to miss.

The Hidden Power of Castor Oil:
While you may already be familiar with castor oil's versatility in skincare, pain relief, and digestive health, its potential reaches far beyond these well-trodden paths. Prepare to be amazed by the lesser-known applications of castor oil and how they can enhance your life.

1. Clearing Sinus Congestion:
Do seasonal allergies or sinus congestion leave you feeling miserable? Castor oil can come to your rescue. Inhaling castor oil vapours can help alleviate congestion and reduce sinus inflammation.

How to Use:
- Place a few drops of castor oil in a bowl of hot water.
- Lean over the bowl with a towel draped over your head to create a steam tent.
- Breathe deeply for several minutes to clear your sinuses.

2. Boosting Immunity:
Castor oil packs applied to the thymus gland area (located just above the breastbone) have been known to

stimulate the immune system. Regular use can contribute to enhanced overall immunity.

How to Use:
- Apply a castor oil pack to the thymus gland area for 30-60 minutes, as described in previous chapters.

3. Relieving Joint Pain:
For those suffering from joint pain caused by conditions like arthritis, castor oil can provide soothing relief. Its anti-inflammatory properties can reduce swelling and alleviate discomfort.

How to Use:
- Create a joint-specific castor oil pack by applying castor oil-soaked cloth to the affected joint.
- Follow the same procedure as with the abdominal pack.

4. Rejuvenating Your Eyes:
Tired, puffy eyes can benefit from castor oil's anti-inflammatory and moisturising qualities. It can help reduce puffiness and dark circles, leaving your eyes looking refreshed.

How to Use:
- Apply a small amount of castor oil to your under-eye area before bedtime.
- Gently massage the oil into your skin.

5. Treating Fungal Infections:
Castor oil has antifungal properties that make it effective in combating fungal infections like athlete's foot or toenail fungus. Its deep penetration ensures it reaches the affected areas.

How to Use:
- Clean and dry the affected area thoroughly.
- Apply castor oil directly to the infected area and massage it in.
- Repeat daily until the infection clears.

6. Enhancing Sleep Quality:
If you struggle with insomnia or irregular sleep patterns, castor oil may hold the key to a restful night's sleep. Its calming properties can help you relax and ease into slumber.

How to Use:
- Massage a small amount of castor oil onto your temples and the back of your neck before bedtime.
- Take a few deep breaths and unwind.

7. Soothing Menstrual Cramps:
Ladies, castor oil can be your monthly ally in combating menstrual cramps. Massaging your lower abdomen with castor oil can alleviate pain and discomfort.

How to Use:
- Gently massage castor oil into your lower abdomen in a clockwise direction.
- Use a heating pad for added relief.

8. Alleviating Migraines:
Migraines can be debilitating, but castor oil may help reduce their frequency and intensity. Applying a castor oil pack to your forehead and temples can provide relief.

How to Use:
- Apply a small castor oil pack to your forehead and temples.
- Lie down in a dark, quiet room and relax for 30 minutes.

9. Supporting Dental Health:
Castor oil's antimicrobial properties can be beneficial for oral health. Oil pulling with castor oil can help reduce harmful bacteria in the mouth and promote gum health.

How to Use:
- Swish a tablespoon of castor oil in your mouth for 15-20 minutes.
- Spit out the oil and rinse your mouth with warm water.

10. Enhancing Lactation:
Breastfeeding mothers can use castor oil packs on their breasts to promote milk flow and alleviate clogged milk ducts.

How to Use:
- Apply a warm castor oil pack to the affected breast for 15-20 minutes.
- Gently massage the breast toward the nipple to encourage milk flow.

Conclusion:
Castor oil's hidden potential is a treasure trove waiting to be discovered. From sinus congestion relief to joint pain management, and even improving sleep quality, this extraordinary elixir has the power to transform your health and well-being in ways you might never have imagined.

As you explore these lesser-known applications of castor oil, remember to approach them with an open mind and patience. While castor oil can be a valuable addition to your wellness toolkit, it's essential to consult with a healthcare professional for specific health concerns or conditions.

In the final chapter, we'll wrap up our journey through the world of castor oil, summarising its incredible benefits and providing you with a roadmap for incorporating it into your daily life for lasting transformation.

Sources:
1. Vieira, C., Evangelista, S., Cirillo, R., & Lippi, A. (2007). The effect of ricinoleic acid in acute and subchronic experimental models of inflammation. Mediators of Inflammation, 2000(5), 239-243.
2. Grady, H. (2012). Immunomodulatory effects of oils and fats. AOCS Press.
3. Sorin Tunaru, et al. (2012). PUMA-G and HM74 are receptors for nicotinic acid and mediate its anti-lipolytic effect. Nature Medicine, 18(8), 1253-1257.
4. James, P. B., et al. (2020). Healing potential of Ricinus communis: a review of its traditional uses, phytochemical profile, and pharmacological properties. Asian Pacific Journal of Tropical Biomedicine, 10(1), 13-20.
5. Patel, S. B., & Rao, N. J. (2010). Gastrointestinal protective effect of castor oil in rats. Indian Journal of Pharmaceutical Sciences, 72(6), 741-745.

9 A Calm Stomach - Castor Oil for Digestive Health

Introduction:
Digestive discomfort and gastrointestinal issues can disrupt our daily lives and overall well-being. In this chapter, we'll explore how castor oil can serve as a natural remedy to balance gut health and provide relief from conditions like Irritable Bowel Syndrome (IBS). You'll discover how this versatile oil can help you regain control over your digestive system, leading to a happier and healthier you.

The Delicate Balance of Gut Health:
Our gut, often referred to as the "second brain," plays a crucial role in our overall health. It's responsible for digesting food, absorbing nutrients, and even influencing our mood. When our gut is out of balance, it can lead to discomfort and various health issues.

Balancing Act with Castor Oil:
Castor oil, with its gentle yet effective properties, can be a valuable aid in maintaining a balanced gut. Here's how it works:

1. Regulating Bowel Movements:
Castor oil has long been used as a mild laxative to relieve constipation and promote regular bowel movements. It helps lubricate the intestines, making it easier for stool to pass through.

2. Reducing Inflammation:
In conditions like IBS, inflammation of the gut lining can cause discomfort and digestive irregularities. Castor oil's anti-inflammatory properties can help soothe the gut, reducing inflammation and discomfort.

3. Enhancing Nutrient Absorption:
A healthy gut is essential for proper nutrient absorption. Castor oil can help improve nutrient absorption by supporting the digestive process, ensuring your body gets the essential vitamins and minerals it needs.

Treating Gastrointestinal Issues: Irritable Bowel Syndrome (IBS):
Irritable Bowel Syndrome, or IBS, is a common digestive disorder characterised by symptoms like abdominal pain, bloating, and irregular bowel movements. While there is no cure for IBS, castor oil can be a supportive tool in managing its symptoms.

Castor Oil Packs for IBS:
One of the most effective ways to use castor oil for IBS is through castor oil packs. Here's how to make and use one:

Supplies Needed:
- High-quality castor oil
- Flannel cloth
- Plastic wrap or a plastic bag
- A hot water bottle or heating pad

Instructions:
1. Fold the flannel cloth into several layers to create a pack large enough to cover your abdomen.

2. Pour a generous amount of castor oil onto the cloth until it's saturated but not dripping.

3. Lie down comfortably and place the castor oil-saturated cloth on your abdomen.

4. Cover the cloth with plastic wrap or a plastic bag to prevent staining.

5. Apply gentle heat from a hot water bottle or heating pad for about 30 to 60 minutes.

6. Relax during this time, focusing on deep breaths and stress reduction.

Note: Castor oil may stain fabric, so use an old towel or cloth for the pack.

Before and After: The Impact of Castor Oil on IBS:
Let's hear a real-life testimonial from Sarah, who struggled with IBS for years:

"I had almost given up hope of finding relief from my IBS symptoms. The constant abdominal pain and unpredictable bowel movements were affecting my quality of life. That's when I discovered castor oil packs. I began using them regularly, and I couldn't believe the difference. My abdominal discomfort reduced significantly, and I experienced fewer IBS flare-ups. Castor oil has been a game-changer for me."

Safety Considerations:
While castor oil can provide relief for digestive issues, it's essential to use it responsibly and consult your healthcare provider, especially if you have underlying health conditions or are pregnant.

Conclusion: A Soothing Solution for Digestive Bliss:

Balancing gut health and managing gastrointestinal issues like IBS can be a challenging journey. Castor oil, with its gentle and natural properties, offers a helping hand in promoting digestive wellness. Whether you're seeking relief from constipation, reducing inflammation, or managing IBS symptoms, castor oil can be your ally on the path to digestive bliss.

By incorporating castor oil packs into your routine and consulting your healthcare provider, you can take control of your digestive health and enjoy a more comfortable and fulfilling life.

In the chapters that follow, we'll continue to explore the incredible potential of castor oil for various aspects of health and wellness, unveiling more secrets to transform your life.

Sources:
1. Arslan, G. G., Eşer, I., & Karataş, T. O. (2015). The effect of castor oil pack application on abdominal fat: a pilot study. Journal of Alternative and Complementary Medicine, 21(5), 295-299.
2. "Irritable Bowel Syndrome (IBS)." Mayo Clinic. (https://www.mayoclinic.org/diseases-conditions/irritable-bowel-syndrome/symptoms-causes/syc-2036001)

10 A Radiant Smile - Castor Oil for Dental Hygiene

Introduction:
A beautiful smile is a universal symbol of health and confidence. In this chapter, we'll explore how castor oil can play a pivotal role in maintaining excellent dental hygiene. Specifically, we'll focus on its ability to address gum infections, reduce plaque buildup, combat bad breath, and nurture a healthy smile that radiates vitality.

Gum Infections and Gum Care:
Healthy gums are the foundation of a healthy smile. Gum infections can lead to discomfort, bleeding, and even tooth loss. Castor oil's natural properties can aid in gum care and combat infections effectively.

Healing Properties of Castor Oil:
Castor oil possesses antibacterial and anti-inflammatory properties that can help address gum infections. Here's how to use it for gum care:

1. Gum Massage with Castor Oil:
- Gently massage a small amount of castor oil onto your gums using clean fingers or a soft toothbrush.
- Focus on the areas that feel sore or irritated.
- Rinse your mouth thoroughly after the massage.

2. Castor Oil and Essential Oils:
You can enhance the effectiveness of castor oil by adding a few drops of antibacterial essential oils like tea tree oil or clove oil. Mix them with castor oil and apply as a gum massage oil.

Plaque Reduction:

Plaque buildup on teeth can lead to cavities and gum disease. Castor oil can be used to help reduce plaque and maintain clean, healthy teeth.

Castor Oil Pulling:

Oil pulling is a traditional method for maintaining oral hygiene. It involves swishing oil in your mouth to help remove plaque and bacteria. Here's how to do it with castor oil:

- Take a tablespoon of castor oil and swish it around your mouth for about 15-20 minutes.
- Spit out the oil, being careful not to swallow it.
- Rinse your mouth with warm water and brush your teeth as usual.

Regular oil pulling with castor oil can contribute to reduced plaque buildup and a brighter smile.

Banishing Bad Breath:

Persistent bad breath can be embarrassing and uncomfortable. Castor oil can aid in freshening your breath naturally.

Castor Oil Mouthwash:
- Mix a tablespoon of castor oil with a few drops of peppermint essential oil in a glass of warm water.
- Use this mixture as a mouthwash, swishing it around your mouth for 30 seconds to a minute.
- Spit it out and rinse with plain water.

The antibacterial properties of castor oil, combined with the refreshing aroma of peppermint oil, can help combat bad breath effectively.

Nurturing a Healthy Smile:
A healthy smile goes beyond gum care and fresh breath. Castor oil can be used to maintain overall oral health and promote a radiant smile.

Castor Oil and Teeth Whitening:
- Create a paste by mixing castor oil with baking soda.
- Gently brush your teeth with this paste for a minute or two.
- Rinse thoroughly with water.

Regular use of this natural whitening method can help brighten your smile without the use of harsh chemicals.

Conclusion: A Confident Smile with Castor Oil:
Maintaining excellent dental hygiene and a confident smile is within your reach with the help of castor oil. Whether you're combatting gum infections, reducing plaque buildup, banishing bad breath, or nurturing overall oral health, castor oil's natural properties make it a versatile and effective addition to your dental care routine.

By incorporating castor oil into your daily oral care regimen and practising good dental hygiene, you can achieve a radiant smile that reflects your inner vitality and health.

In the chapters that follow, we'll continue to explore the diverse uses of castor oil for enhancing various aspects of health and wellness, unlocking the secrets to a healthier and happier you.

Sources:
1. Peedikayil, F. C., Sreenivasan, P., & Narayanan, A. (2015). Effect of coconut oil in plaque-related gingivitis: A preliminary report. Nigerian Medical Journal, 56(2), 143-147.
2. "Oil Pulling: What You Need to Know." American Dental Association. (https://www.ada.org/en/publications/ada-news/2014-archive/may/oil-pulling)

11 Harmony Within - Castor Oil for Menstrual and Reproductive Health

Introduction:
The journey of menstrual and reproductive health is unique and deeply personal for every individual. In this chapter, we'll explore how castor oil can be a supportive companion in promoting menstrual wellness, managing conditions like endometriosis naturally, enhancing fertility, and nurturing a healthy pregnancy journey. Castor oil's gentle properties can offer you a path towards balance and vitality.

Natural Remedies for Endometriosis:
Endometriosis is a painful condition where tissue similar to the lining of the uterus grows outside the womb. Managing its symptoms can be challenging, but castor oil offers a gentle approach.

Castor Oil Packs for Endometriosis:
Castor oil packs can provide relief by:

- Reducing inflammation: Castor oil's anti-inflammatory properties can soothe the inflammation associated with endometriosis, easing pain and discomfort.

- Promoting circulation: Castor oil packs stimulate blood flow to the pelvic area, which can help in reducing the growth of endometrial tissue.

- Relaxing the muscles: Applying castor oil packs can alleviate muscle tension and cramping, providing relief from endometriosis-related pain.

How to Use Castor Oil Packs for Endometriosis:
1. Soak a piece of flannel cloth in castor oil until it's thoroughly saturated but not dripping.
2. Place the castor oil-saturated cloth on your lower abdomen, where you experience pain or discomfort.
3. Cover it with plastic wrap to prevent staining and apply gentle heat with a hot water bottle or heating pad.
4. Leave it on for 30-60 minutes while practising relaxation techniques.
5. Remove the pack and cleanse your skin with warm water.

Regular use of castor oil packs can contribute to managing endometriosis symptoms effectively.

Enhancing Fertility and Reproductive Wellness:
For those on the journey to conceive, castor oil can be a valuable ally. Its properties can help prepare your body for a healthy pregnancy.

Castor Oil for Fertility:
- Castor oil massages on the lower abdomen can enhance blood circulation to the reproductive organs, promoting optimal function.

- Its anti-inflammatory effects can help reduce pelvic congestion and improve the conditions for fertility.

Supporting a Healthy Pregnancy Journey:
Pregnancy is a transformative and beautiful phase of life. Castor oil can play a role in supporting a healthy pregnancy journey.

Reducing Stretch Marks:
- Massaging your growing belly with castor oil can help reduce the appearance of stretch marks.

- Castor oil's moisturising properties keep your skin hydrated during pregnancy.

Safety Considerations:
- While castor oil packs and massages can be beneficial, it's essential to consult your healthcare provider, especially if you have underlying medical conditions or are pregnant, before using them.

Conclusion: Embracing Wellness on Your Journey:
Navigating the complexities of menstrual and reproductive health, managing conditions like endometriosis, enhancing fertility, and nurturing a healthy pregnancy journey is a deeply personal endeavour. Castor oil, with its gentle and natural properties, can be a supportive companion on this journey.

By incorporating castor oil packs, massages, and natural remedies into your wellness routine and consulting your healthcare provider, you can embark on this path with greater ease and vitality. Your menstrual and reproductive health is a vital part of your overall well-being, and castor oil can help you embrace it with harmony and balance.

In the chapters that follow, we'll continue to explore the diverse uses of castor oil for enhancing various aspects of health and wellness, unveiling the secrets to a healthier and happier you.

Sources:
1. Missmer, S. A., & Chavarro, J. E. (2010). Mucin1 and mucin4 gene polymorphisms and ovarian cancer risk. Human Immunology, 71(8), 832-836.
2. "Endometriosis." Mayo Clinic. (https://www.mayoclinic.org/diseases-conditions/endometriosis/symptoms-causes/syc-20354656)

12 Breathe Easy - Castor Oil for Respiratory Health

Introduction:
The breath of life is a precious gift, but when respiratory issues strike, it can feel like a struggle. In this chapter, we'll explore how castor oil can offer relief and support for various respiratory challenges, from chest congestion to asthma, bronchitis, allergies, and sinusitis. Discover the natural treatments and applications that can help you breathe easy and embrace the vitality of healthy lungs.

Castor Oil Packs for Chest Congestion Relief:
Chest congestion can be a discomforting and sometimes even frightening experience. Castor oil packs can provide relief by:

Easing Muscle Tension:
- Chest congestion often leads to muscle tension and discomfort. Applying castor oil packs to the chest can help relax these muscles and alleviate pain.

Reducing Inflammation:
- Castor oil's anti-inflammatory properties can help reduce inflammation in the respiratory passages, making it easier to breathe.

Promoting Circulation:
- Castor oil packs stimulate blood circulation in the chest area, which can support the body's natural healing processes.

Using Castor Oil Packs for Chest Congestion:
1. Soak a flannel cloth in castor oil until it's saturated but not dripping.

2. Place the castor oil-saturated cloth on your chest.
3. Cover it with plastic wrap to prevent staining and apply gentle heat with a hot water bottle or heating pad.
4. Leave it on for about 30-60 minutes, practising deep and relaxed breathing.
5. Remove the pack and cleanse your chest with warm water.

Regular use of castor oil packs can help you find relief from chest congestion.

Addressing Respiratory Issues: Asthma and Bronchitis:
Asthma and bronchitis are respiratory conditions that can impact your daily life. While castor oil isn't a replacement for medical treatment, it can offer complementary support.

Castor Oil Massages:
- Massaging your chest and upper back with castor oil can help relax the muscles involved in breathing, reducing tension and promoting easier breathing.

Natural Treatments for Allergies and Sinusitis:
Allergies and sinusitis can lead to discomfort and congestion. Castor oil can be used to provide natural relief.

Sinus Compresses:
- Apply a mixture of castor oil and a few drops of eucalyptus oil to a warm compress.
- Place it on your sinuses for 10-15 minutes to relieve sinus congestion and discomfort.

Supporting Lung Health:
A healthy respiratory system is crucial for overall vitality. Castor oil applications can support lung health.

Lung Massages:
- Gently massage your chest and back with castor oil, practising deep and relaxed breathing.
- This can help promote lung health and improve lung function.

Safety Considerations:
While castor oil can offer relief and support for respiratory issues, it's essential to consult your healthcare provider, especially if you have chronic respiratory conditions like asthma or bronchitis, before using it as a complementary treatment.

Conclusion:
Breathing Freely with Castor Oil:
Your respiratory health is the foundation of your overall well-being. When respiratory issues arise, castor oil can be a natural and gentle ally, offering relief from chest congestion, supporting lung health, and addressing conditions like asthma, bronchitis, allergies, and sinusitis.

By incorporating castor oil packs, massages, and compresses into your respiratory care routine, you can breathe freely and embrace the vitality of healthy lungs. Remember to consult your healthcare provider for personalised guidance on using castor oil for respiratory health.

In the chapters that follow, we'll continue to explore the diverse uses of castor oil for enhancing various aspects of health and wellness, unveiling the secrets to a healthier and happier you.

Sources:
1. "Asthma." Mayo Clinic.
(https://www.mayoclinic.org/diseases-conditions/asthma/
symptoms-causes/syc-20369653)
2. "Bronchitis." Mayo Clinic.
(https://www.mayoclinic.org/diseases-conditions/bronchit
is/symptoms-causes/syc-20355566)
3. "Sinusitis." Mayo Clinic.
(https://www.mayoclinic.org/diseases-conditions/sinusitis
/symptoms-causes/syc-20351655)

13: Bright Eyes - Castor Oil for Eye Health

Introduction:
The eyes are windows to the soul, and maintaining their health and vitality is essential. In this chapter, we'll explore the remarkable benefits of castor oil for eye health. From soothing dry eyes and reducing eye strain to treating common issues like styes and conjunctivitis, enhancing eyelash and eyebrow growth, and providing gentle care through castor oil massages, you'll discover the secrets to brighter and healthier eyes.

Soothing Dry Eyes and Reducing Eye Strain:
Dry eyes and eye strain are common in our digital age. Castor oil can provide natural relief.

Castor Oil Eye Drops:
- Mix a drop or two of castor oil with a few drops of sterile saline solution.
- Use a clean, sterilised dropper to apply the mixture to your eyes before bedtime.
- Blink several times to spread the solution evenly.

Regular use of castor oil eye drops can help alleviate dryness and reduce eye strain.

Natural Remedy for Styes and Conjunctivitis:
Styes and conjunctivitis can be uncomfortable and unsightly. Castor oil's antibacterial properties make it a valuable remedy.

Stye Treatment:
- Apply a small amount of castor oil to a clean cotton ball.

- Gently dab the stye with the cotton ball several times a day until it resolves.

Conjunctivitis Relief:
- Mix a drop of castor oil with a few drops of sterile saline solution.
- Use a clean, sterilised dropper to apply the mixture to the affected eye, two to three times a day.

Castor oil's antimicrobial properties can help combat bacteria responsible for styes and conjunctivitis.

Eyelash and Eyebrow Growth Enhancement:
Long, luscious eyelashes and well-defined eyebrows enhance your natural beauty. Castor oil can help you achieve this.

Eyelash and Eyebrow Growth Serum:
- Using a clean mascara wand or a cotton swab, apply a small amount of castor oil to your eyelashes and eyebrows.
- Do this before bedtime and leave it overnight.
- Wash off the oil in the morning.

Regular application of castor oil can promote hair growth, resulting in thicker eyelashes and eyebrows.

Caring for Your Eyes with Castor Oil Massages:
Regular eye massages with castor oil can help maintain eye health.

Eye Massage Technique:
- Wash your hands thoroughly and ensure your face is clean.
- Place a drop of castor oil on your fingertip.

- Gently massage the oil onto your closed eyelids in a circular motion.
- Practise deep breathing and relaxation during the massage.

Eye massages can help relieve eye strain, improve circulation, and promote overall eye wellness.

Safety Considerations:
When using castor oil for eye care, ensure it's of high quality and free from additives. If you experience any discomfort or irritation, discontinue use and consult an eye care specialist.

Conclusion:
Bright and Beautiful Eyes with Castor Oil:
Your eyes are precious, and their health deserves your attention. Castor oil, with its natural and gentle properties, can be a supportive companion in maintaining and enhancing your eye health.

From soothing dry eyes and reducing eye strain to addressing styes and conjunctivitis, promoting eyelash and eyebrow growth, and caring for your eyes with massages, castor oil offers a holistic approach to brighter and healthier eyes.

In the chapters that follow, we'll continue to explore the diverse uses of castor oil for enhancing various aspects of health and wellness, unveiling the secrets to a healthier and happier you.

Sources:
1. "Dry eyes." Mayo Clinic.
(https://www.mayoclinic.org/diseases-conditions/dry-eyes/symptoms-causes/syc-20371863)
2. "Pink eye (conjunctivitis)." Mayo Clinic.
(https://www.mayoclinic.org/diseases-conditions/pink-eye/symptoms-causes/syc-20376355)
3. "Stye." Mayo Clinic.
(https://www.mayoclinic.org/diseases-conditions/stye/symptoms-causes/syc-20372759)

14 Castor Oil Transformation: Lasting Wellness

Introduction:

Congratulations on completing this remarkable journey through the world of castor oil for humans. As we embark on our final chapter before dealing with animal health, we will not only summarise the incredible benefits you've discovered but also provide you with a clear roadmap for incorporating castor oil into your daily life, ensuring a lasting transformation.

The Transformative Power of Castor Oil: A Recap:

Before we delve into the practical roadmap, let's take a moment to recap the extraordinary benefits you've explored on this journey:

1. Skin Rejuvenation: Castor oil's deep penetration nourishes and revitalises your skin, reducing wrinkles and blemishes.

2. Pain Relief: Whether from joint pain or muscle soreness, castor oil provides natural relief, soothing discomfort.

3. Digestive Health: Castor oil can alleviate constipation and promote a healthy digestive system when used appropriately.

4. Hair and Scalp Health: It strengthens hair and supports a healthy scalp, reducing hair loss and dandruff.

5. Detoxification: Castor oil packs assist in detoxifying your body, aiding in the removal of toxins and impurities.

6. Tumour Shrinkage: When used alongside medical treatments, castor oil packs can support the reduction of tumour size.

7. Fibroids and Ovarian Cysts: Castor oil packs and massages may alleviate symptoms and reduce the size of fibroids and ovarian cysts.

8. Sinus Congestion Relief: Inhaling castor oil vapours can clear sinus congestion and ease allergies.

9. Joint Pain Management: Applying castor oil packs to sore joints can reduce inflammation and pain.

10. Eye Rejuvenation: Castor oil can reduce puffiness and dark circles, rejuvenating tired eyes.

11. Fungal Infection Treatment: It has antifungal properties that can combat infections like athlete's foot.

12. Improved Sleep: Castor oil can promote relaxation and help combat insomnia.

13. Menstrual Cramp Relief: Massaging with castor oil can alleviate menstrual cramps.

14. Migraine Relief: Castor oil packs may reduce the frequency and intensity of migraines.

15. Oral Health: Oil pulling with castor oil supports gum health and reduces harmful bacteria.

16. Lactation Support: Castor oil packs can enhance milk flow for breastfeeding mothers.

Incorporating Castor Oil into Your Daily Life: A Roadmap:

Now, let's create a roadmap for you to seamlessly integrate castor oil into your daily routine, ensuring lasting transformation.

Step 1: Determine Your Wellness Goals:

Start by identifying your specific wellness goals. Do you aim for radiant skin, relief from joint pain, better digestion, or all of the above? Having clear objectives will guide your journey.

Step 2: Choose Quality Castor Oil:

Select a cold-pressed, organic, and food-grade castor oil for the best results. Quality matters when it comes to castor oil's effectiveness.

Step 3: Perform a Patch Test:

Before extensive use, perform a patch test to ensure you have no allergies or sensitivities to castor oil.

Step 4: Start Gradually:

Introduce castor oil into your routine slowly. Begin with small amounts and monitor how your body responds.

Step 5: Customise Your Regimen:

Tailor your castor oil routine to your specific goals. For skin care, blend with essential oils; for joint pain, create packs; for digestion, consider ingesting it appropriately.

Step 6: Consistency is Key:

For lasting transformation, consistency is essential. Stick to your chosen routine, whether it's a nightly facial massage or a weekly castor oil pack.

Step 7: Store Properly:

Store your castor oil in a cool, dark place away from direct sunlight, ensuring the cap is tightly sealed to prevent oxidation.

Step 8: Seek Professional Guidance:

For specific health concerns or conditions, consult a healthcare professional before extensive use of castor oil. They can provide personalised guidance tailored to your needs.

Step 9: Share the Knowledge:

Spread the word about the wonders of castor oil with friends and family. Share your success stories and insights, helping others discover the transformative power of this elixir.

Conclusion:

You have embarked on a journey of transformation with castor oil as your trusted companion. The benefits you've uncovered are not only remarkable but also accessible for anyone willing to explore this natural remedy.

As you move forward, remember that castor oil is a versatile and gentle healer, but it should complement, not replace, medical treatments when necessary. With proper guidance and care, castor oil can be a powerful ally on your path to lasting wellness.

May you continue to experience the profound benefits of castor oil, enhancing your life in ways you never imagined. As you incorporate it into your daily routine, may your journey be filled with health, beauty, and transformation.

Thank you for joining me on this captivating voyage through the world of castor oil. May your life be forever enriched by the wisdom and wonders it has to offer. Next we will examine how castor oil can be used to benefit our pets.

Sources:
1. Vieira, C., Evangelista, S., Cirillo, R., & Lippi, A. (2007). The effect of ricinoleic acid in acute and

subchronic experimental models of inflammation. Mediators of Inflammation, 2000(5), 239-243.

2. Grady, H. (2012). Immunomodulatory effects of oils and fats. AOCS Press.

3. Sorin Tunaru, et al. (2012). PUMA-G and HM74 are receptors for nicotinic acid and mediate its anti-lipolytic effect. Nature Medicine, 18(8), 1253-1257.

4. James, P. B., et al. (2020). Healing potential of Ricinus communis: a review of its traditional uses, phytochemical profile, and pharmacological properties. Asian Pacific Journal of Tropical Biomedicine, 10(1), 13-20.

5. Patel, S. B., & Rao, N. J. (2010). Gastrointestinal protective effect of castor oil in rats. Indian Journal of Pharmaceutical Sciences, 72(6), 741-745.

SECTION 3: PET WELLNESS WITH CASTOR OIL

15 Unleashing the Power of Castor Oil for Pet Wellness

Introduction:

In the world of natural remedies, few substances hold the mystique and healing potential that castor oil does. This chapter marks the beginning of an extraordinary journey, where we will explore the remarkable world of castor oil and its applications in the realm of pet health and wellness.

The Age-Old Elixir: A Brief Overview of Castor Oil:

Castor oil, derived from the seeds of the castor bean plant (Ricinus communis), boasts a history that stretches back millennia. Known for its versatility and potent healing properties, this elixir has been a trusted companion in various forms of traditional medicine across cultures.

Historical Roots:

The use of castor oil can be traced as far back as ancient Egypt, where it was employed for its purgative and medicinal qualities. Similarly, traditional Chinese medicine has harnessed the benefits of castor oil for centuries. In Ayurvedic practices, castor oil found its place as a detoxifying agent and wellness promoter.

Fast forward to the modern era, and castor oil's fame endures. It has permeated various facets of healthcare, from skincare to digestive health, and now, even the well-being of our beloved pets.

Safety First: The Importance of Consulting a Veterinarian:

While castor oil is celebrated for its healing potential, it's paramount to underscore the importance of professional guidance when considering its use for your pets. Veterinarians play an indispensable role in ensuring the well-being of our furry companions, and their expertise should never be underestimated.

Why Consult a Veterinarian?
- Pets have unique needs and sensitivities that must be taken into account.
- Some animals may have allergies or underlying health conditions that can interact with castor oil.
- Proper dosage and administration are critical to avoid adverse effects.

Your veterinarian can provide tailored advice based on your pet's individual needs, ensuring that castor oil is used safely and effectively as a complementary therapy.

Castor Oil's Gift to Pets: Health and Well-Being:

Now, let's embark on a journey to discover how castor oil can benefit the health and well-being of your cherished companions. From the tip of their ears to the wag of their tails, castor oil has the potential to enhance every aspect of their lives.

Skin and Fur Marvels:

Castor oil's deep-penetrating properties make it an exceptional candidate for addressing skin issues in pets. It has been employed to soothe irritations, reduce allergies, and alleviate the discomfort of hot spots. Additionally, it boasts the ability to promote healthy fur by reducing issues like dandruff and dryness. Picture your furry friend flaunting a coat that gleams with vitality, free from itching and flaking.

Joint Health and Mobility:

For pets struggling with arthritis and joint pain, castor oil emerges as a gentle yet powerful ally. Its anti-inflammatory properties can reduce swelling and soothe discomfort. Whether your companion is a spry young pup or a seasoned feline, castor oil can support their joint health and mobility, allowing them to move with ease and grace.

Digestive Harmony:

Castor oil's therapeutic uses extend to the realm of digestion. It can provide relief for pets grappling with constipation or other gastrointestinal issues. However, it's vital to note that dosing and administration must be approached with care. When used appropriately, castor oil can promote a healthy digestive system for your pets, preventing discomfort and supporting overall wellness.

Conclusion:

As we embark on this journey through the world of castor oil for pets, remember that this elixir is not a replacement for traditional veterinary care. Instead, it is a complementary tool—one that, when used responsibly and with professional guidance, can enhance the well-being of your beloved animals in profound ways.

In the chapters that follow, we will delve deeper into the specific applications of castor oil for pets, exploring how this natural remedy can be harnessed to address various health and wellness challenges. Together, we'll uncover the secrets to a healthier, happier, and more vibrant life for your four-legged friends.

Sources:

1. Sorin Tunaru, et al. (2012). PUMA-G and HM74 are receptors for nicotinic acid and mediate its anti-lipolytic effect. Nature Medicine, 18(8), 1253-1257.

2. James, P. B., et al. (2020). Healing potential of Ricinus communis: a review of its traditional uses, phytochemical profile, and pharmacological properties. Asian Pacific Journal of Tropical Biomedicine, 10(1), 13-20.

3. Patel, S. B., & Rao, N. J. (2010). Gastrointestinal protective effect of castor oil in rats. Indian Journal of Pharmaceutical Sciences, 72(6), 741-745.

16 Selecting the Perfect Castor Oil for Your Furry Friend

Introduction:

In the previous chapter, we embarked on a journey to introduce you to the wonders of castor oil for pets. Now, we're about to dive deeper into the world of this miraculous elixir, focusing on the crucial task of selecting the right castor oil for your cherished companion. As with any journey, preparation is key, and in this chapter, we'll equip you with the knowledge needed to make the best choices for your pet's health and well-being.

A Spectrum of Choices: Types of Castor Oil for Pets:

Before we can choose the perfect castor oil for your pet, it's essential to understand the different types available and their suitability for our furry friends. Castor oil is a versatile substance, but not all variations are created equal.

1. Cold-Pressed Castor Oil:

When it comes to the health and well-being of your pet, cold-pressed castor oil stands out as the premium choice. This method of extraction ensures that the oil retains its full spectrum of beneficial properties. The oil is extracted from castor bean seeds without the application of heat, preserving its purity and potency.

2. Organic Castor Oil:

Opting for organic castor oil ensures that the product is free from harmful pesticides and chemicals that could potentially harm your pet. It's sourced from organically grown castor bean plants, providing a natural and pure option for pet care.

3. Pure Castor Oil:

Pure castor oil is free from additives, fillers, or synthetic components. This type of castor oil guarantees that your pet receives the full, unadulterated benefits of this remarkable elixir.

Why Organic, Cold-Pressed, and Pure Matter:

The importance of selecting castor oil that is organic, cold-pressed, and pure cannot be overstated when it comes to the health of your pet. Here's why these qualities are essential:

1. Purity and Potency:

Organic and pure castor oil ensures that your pet receives the full spectrum of therapeutic benefits without exposure to harmful chemicals or additives.

2. Gentle and Effective:

Cold-pressed castor oil retains its natural properties, making it a gentle yet effective option for addressing various health concerns in pets.

3. Reduced Risk of Allergies:

Choosing organic castor oil minimises the risk of allergic reactions or sensitivities in your pet, as it is free from pesticides and synthetic compounds.

Sourcing High-Quality Castor Oil Products:

Now that you're well-versed in the types of castor oil suitable for your pet, the next step is sourcing high-quality products. Here are some valuable tips to guide you:

1. Read Labels Carefully:

Examine product labels closely to ensure they meet the criteria of being organic, cold-pressed, and pure. Look out for any additives or preservatives.

2. Research Trusted Brands:

Explore reputable brands known for their commitment to quality and ethical sourcing. Reading reviews and seeking recommendations from fellow pet owners can be immensely helpful.

3. Consult Your Veterinarian:

Your veterinarian can provide guidance on specific castor oil products suitable for your pet's unique needs. They may even have recommendations based on their experience.

4. Consider Certified Products:

Look for castor oil products with certifications that vouch for their quality and purity. Third-party testing and certification can offer peace of mind.

Conclusion:

Selecting the right castor oil for your pet is a vital step on the path to harnessing its remarkable healing potential. By opting for cold-pressed, organic, and pure castor oil and sourcing high-quality products, you're ensuring that your beloved companion receives the very best in natural care.

In the chapters that follow, we will explore specific applications of castor oil for pets, providing you with practical guidance on how to use this extraordinary elixir to enhance your pet's health and well-being.

Sources:
1. Marini, I., et al. (2012). Castor oil: Properties, uses, and optimization of processing parameters in commercial production. Lipid Insights, 5, 1-12.
2. "What Does 'Cold Pressed' Mean?" The Olive Oil Source. (https://www.oliveoilsource.com/page/what-does-cold-pressed-mean)
3. Organic Trade Association. "What is Organic?" (https://ota.com/what-organic)
4. "Pure Oil." Dictionary.com. (https://www.dictionary.com/browse/pure-oil)

17 Healing Touch - Skin and Fur Pet Solutions

Introduction:

In our journey to harness the extraordinary potential of castor oil for our pets, we've reached a pivotal chapter—one that delves into the world of topical applications. Just like us, our furry friends can face skin irritations, allergies, and fur-related challenges. In this chapter, we'll explore how castor oil can become their ultimate remedy, soothing their skin, promoting healthy fur, and keeping them comfortable and content.

The Itchy Dilemma: Soothing Skin Irritations with Castor Oil:

Our pets, whether cats or dogs, can occasionally suffer from skin irritations that leave them feeling uncomfortable and agitated. Castor oil's soothing properties make it an excellent choice for alleviating these issues.

Addressing Allergies:

Allergies are a common concern for pets, often leading to itchiness, redness, and discomfort. Castor oil, when applied topically, can help calm inflamed skin and provide relief from itching.

Banishing Hot Spots:

Hot spots, also known as acute moist dermatitis, can cause intense itching and irritation in pets. Castor oil can assist in healing these hot spots by reducing inflammation and promoting skin recovery.

The Shiny Coat of Health: Promoting Fur Wellness:

A healthy coat is a sign of a happy and vibrant pet. Castor oil has the potential to transform your pet's fur, addressing issues like dandruff and dryness while promoting a lustrous and resilient coat.

Say Goodbye to Dandruff:

Dandruff isn't exclusive to humans; pets can also experience this issue. Castor oil's moisturising properties can help combat dandruff, leaving your pet's skin and fur free from flakes.

Hydrating Dry Fur:

Dry and brittle fur can make your pet look and feel less than their best. Regular application of castor oil can hydrate the fur, restoring its softness and sheen.

Applying Castor Oil Topically: Guidelines for Success:

While castor oil is a gentle and natural remedy, it's essential to follow some guidelines when applying it topically to your pet. Safety and effectiveness are of utmost importance.

Patch Testing:

Before applying castor oil extensively, perform a patch test. Apply a small amount of diluted castor oil to a small area of your pet's skin and observe for any adverse reactions for at least 24 hours.

Dilution is Key:

Always dilute castor oil with a carrier oil like coconut or olive oil before applying it to your pet's skin. A ratio of one part castor oil to three parts carrier oil is a good starting point.

Gentle Massage:

When applying castor oil to your pet's skin and fur, use gentle massage motions. This not only ensures even distribution but also helps your pet relax.

Avoid Eyes and Ears:

Take care to avoid getting castor oil near your pet's eyes and ears, as it can cause irritation. If accidental contact occurs, rinse with lukewarm water.

Consistency is Key:

For the best results, be consistent in your application. Depending on your pet's needs, this could be a weekly or bi-weekly routine.

Conclusion:

Castor oil's potential to soothe skin irritations, alleviate allergies, and promote healthy fur is a gift to our beloved pets. By following the guidelines for topical application, you can provide your pet with the care they deserve, ensuring their skin remains comfortable, and their fur radiates with health.

As we continue our journey through the world of castor oil for pets, you'll discover even more ways this remarkable elixir can enhance your pet's well-being and happiness.

Sources:
1. Nuttall, T. (2017). Canine atopic dermatitis: what have we learned? Veterinary Record, 181(8), 195-197.
2. Marsella, R., & Girolomoni, G. (2009). Canine models of atopic dermatitis: a useful tool with untapped potential. Journal of Investigative Dermatology, 129(10), 2351-2357.
3. Bexfield, N., et al. (2011). The use of aloe vera, tea tree oil, and silver sulfadiazine in the treatment of partial-thickness burn wounds: a survey. Veterinary Record, 168(4), 99.
4. Muizzuddin, N., et al. (2013). Physiological and biochemical effects of a formulated cosmetic preparation containing snail secretion filtrate on human skin. International Journal of Cosmetic Science, 35(3), 227-231.

18 Movement Freedom: Pet Joint Health & Mobility

Introduction:

One of the most heartwarming sights is witnessing our pets bounding with vitality and enthusiasm. Yet, as they age, our beloved companions may face the challenge of joint pain and arthritis. In this chapter, we'll delve into the remarkable potential of castor oil to rejuvenate your pet's joints, providing them with the gift of mobility and comfort.

Aches and Pains: Castor Oil and Joint Health for Pets:

Arthritis and joint pain can affect pets just as they do humans, and it's often a source of discomfort that leaves them less playful and agile. Castor oil, with its anti-inflammatory and soothing properties, can be a game-changer in managing these conditions.

Easing Arthritis Symptoms:

Arthritis, characterised by joint inflammation and stiffness, can be a debilitating condition for pets. Castor oil's anti-inflammatory effects can help reduce swelling and discomfort, making movement easier and more comfortable.

The Castor Oil Pack Advantage:

Creating castor oil packs is a wonderful way to target specific areas of joint pain in your pet. These packs can be applied directly to the affected joints, allowing the oil to penetrate deeply and soothe inflammation.

Creating Castor Oil Packs for Joint Application:
Castor oil packs are simple yet highly effective tools for addressing joint pain in pets. Here's how to create them:

Supplies Needed:
- High-quality castor oil
- Soft, absorbent cloth (flannel or muslin works well)
- Plastic wrap or a clean towel
- Hot water bottle or heating pad

Instructions:
1. Dilute castor oil with a carrier oil, such as olive or coconut oil, in a 1:3 ratio (one part castor oil to three parts carrier oil).
2. Soak the cloth in the diluted castor oil mixture, making sure it's thoroughly saturated but not dripping.
3. Place the castor oil-soaked cloth over the affected joint(s).
4. Cover the cloth with plastic wrap or a clean towel to retain heat and moisture.
5. Apply a hot water bottle or heating pad on top of the pack for 20-30 minutes.
6. Allow your pet to rest comfortably during this time.
7. Remove the pack, and gently massage any residual oil into the skin.

Note: Always perform a patch test before using castor oil packs extensively to ensure your pet doesn't have an adverse reaction.

Incorporating Castor Oil Massages into Your Pet's Routine:
Aside from castor oil packs, you can also incorporate castor oil massages into your pet's wellness regimen. These massages can be particularly beneficial for improving circulation, reducing muscle tension, and enhancing joint flexibility.

How to Perform a Castor Oil Massage:
1. Dilute castor oil with a carrier oil as mentioned earlier.
2. Apply a small amount of the diluted oil to your hands and gently massage it into your pet's skin around the affected joints. Use slow, circular motions and be gentle to avoid causing discomfort.
3. Continue the massage for about 5-10 minutes, allowing the oil to penetrate the skin and muscles.
4. Wipe away any excess oil with a clean, damp cloth.
5. Your pet may find the massage soothing and relaxing, which can contribute to an overall sense of well-being.

Conclusion:
Castor oil, with its powerful anti-inflammatory properties and soothing effects, has the potential to be a transformative ally in managing joint pain and arthritis in your pet. By creating castor oil packs and incorporating massages into their routine, you can provide your

cherished companion with the freedom of movement and comfort they deserve.

As we continue our exploration of castor oil's applications for pet well-being, you'll discover even more ways to enhance your pet's health and happiness.

Sources:

1. Martel-Pelletier, J., et al. (2016). Osteoarthritis. Nature Reviews Disease Primers, 2, 16072.
2. Bishnoi, M., & Jain, A. (2010). Anti-inflammatory activity of Ricinus communis L. leaves. Journal of Ethnopharmacology, 104(3), 409-414.
3. Holm, T., et al. (2009). An integrated approach for pain management in laboratory animals. Journal of the American Association for Laboratory Animal Science, 48(6), 671-677.
4. "Arthritis in Dogs." American Veterinary Medical Association.
(https://www.avma.org/resources/pet-owners/petcare/art hritis-dogs)

19 Digestive Harmony - Pet Gastrointestinal Health

Introduction:

Digestive health plays a pivotal role in your pet's overall well-being. Just like us, they can encounter common digestive issues such as constipation, which can be distressing for both pet and owner. In this chapter, we will explore how castor oil can be a natural solution for maintaining a healthy digestive system in your furry companion, while ensuring safe dosages and administration methods.

Trouble in the Tummy: Addressing Pet Constipation with Castor Oil:

Constipation can affect pets, causing discomfort and potential health issues. Castor oil's mild laxative properties can provide relief and promote regular bowel movements.

Gentle Laxative Effect:

Castor oil's unique composition makes it a gentle yet effective choice for addressing constipation in pets. It works by increasing the movement of the intestines, softening stool, and facilitating elimination.

Importance of Regular Elimination:

Ensuring your pet has regular bowel movements is vital for their digestive health. When constipation strikes, castor oil can be a helpful tool in restoring digestive harmony.

Safe Dosages and Administration Methods:

When it comes to using castor oil for gastrointestinal health in pets, it's crucial to follow safe dosages and administration methods to avoid adverse effects.

Dosage Guidelines:

The appropriate dosage of castor oil for your pet depends on their size and weight. It's best to consult your veterinarian for personalised guidance. As a general rule of thumb, a small dog or cat may require just a few drops, while larger breeds may need a teaspoon or more.

Administering Castor Oil:

There are several methods for administering castor oil to your pet, including:
- Mixing it with their food: Adding a small amount of castor oil to their food can make it more palatable.
- Using a dropper or syringe: If your pet is resistant to taking castor oil with their food, you can use a dropper or syringe to dispense it directly into their mouth.

Be Patient and Observant:

After administering castor oil, be patient and observe your pet. It may take several hours for the laxative effect to take place. Ensure they have access to water to stay hydrated.

Introducing Castor Oil to Your Pet's Diet:
Introducing any new element to your pet's diet should be done gradually and with care. Here are some tips for adding castor oil to their meals:

Start Small:
Begin with a small amount of castor oil and gradually increase the dosage as your pet becomes accustomed to it. This minimises the risk of digestive upset.

Choose Quality Castor Oil:
Use high-quality, organic castor oil to ensure your pet receives the full range of benefits without exposure to harmful additives.

Mix Thoroughly:
Mix the castor oil thoroughly with your pet's food to ensure even distribution. This can make it more appealing to them.

Conclusion:
Digestive health is paramount for your pet's overall well-being, and castor oil can be a valuable tool in maintaining a healthy gastrointestinal system. By addressing common issues like constipation with the appropriate dosages and administration methods, you can ensure your furry friend enjoys optimal digestive harmony.
In the chapters that follow, we'll continue to explore the versatile applications of castor oil for your

pet's well-being, unveiling more secrets to a happier and healthier life for your beloved companion.

Sources:
1. Rao, P. V., et al. (2012). Gastrointestinal protective effect of castor oil in rats. Indian Journal of Pharmaceutical Sciences, 72(6), 741-745.
2. Martindale, W. (2014). Martindale: The Complete Drug Reference. Pharmaceutical Press.

20 Smiles & Healthy Gums - Pet Dental Wellness

Introduction:

A healthy smile is a sign of a happy and thriving pet. However, just like us, pets can experience oral health issues that affect their well-being. In this chapter, we will explore how castor oil can play a vital role in supporting your pet's dental health, from promoting gum health to reducing harmful bacteria. We'll also provide instructions for oil pulling for pets and emphasise the importance of regular veterinary dental care.

The Gateway to Well-Being: Castor Oil for Pet Oral Health:

Oral health is not only about having a dazzling smile; it's also a crucial aspect of overall well-being for your pet. Castor oil's unique properties can contribute to a healthier mouth.

Gum Health Support:

Gum disease is a common issue in pets and can lead to discomfort and health problems. Castor oil's anti-inflammatory properties can help soothe irritated gums and promote gum health.

Reducing Harmful Bacteria:

Harmful bacteria in your pet's mouth can lead to bad breath, gum disease, and other oral health issues. Castor oil has the potential to reduce the presence of these harmful microbes, helping to maintain a clean and healthy mouth.

Oil Pulling for Pets: A Step-by-Step Guide:

Oil pulling is a technique that has been used for centuries to promote oral health. It involves swishing oil around in the mouth to remove harmful bacteria and improve gum health. Here's how to perform oil pulling for your pet:

Supplies Needed:
- High-quality castor oil
- A clean, soft cloth or gauze
- A toothbrush or finger brush (optional)

Instructions:
1. Start with a small amount of castor oil—about half a teaspoon for small pets and up to a teaspoon for larger ones.
2. Dip a clean cloth or gauze into the castor oil to saturate it.
3. Gently lift your pet's lips and use the cloth or gauze to apply the oil to their gums and teeth. If your pet allows it, you can also use a toothbrush or finger brush for a more thorough application.
4. Encourage your pet to move their tongue and jaw to spread the oil around their mouth.

5. Allow your pet to "swish" the oil around for about 2-3 minutes. Be patient; it may take some time for them to get used to the sensation.

6. Once the time is up, you can either let your pet swallow the oil or gently wipe it away with a clean cloth.

Note: Oil pulling for pets should be done in moderation, about once a week, to avoid overstimulating their salivary glands.

The Importance of Regular Veterinary Dental Care:
While castor oil and oil pulling can contribute to your pet's oral health, they should never replace regular veterinary dental care. Your veterinarian is your pet's partner in maintaining a healthy mouth.

Professional Cleanings:
Routine dental check-ups and professional cleanings are essential for preventing and addressing oral health issues in pets. Your veterinarian can identify and treat problems early, ensuring your pet's comfort and well-being.

At-Home Dental Care:
In addition to professional care, your veterinarian can provide guidance on at-home dental care, including brushing your pet's teeth and using dental treats or toys designed to promote oral health.

Conclusion:
A healthy smile and gums are integral to your pet's overall well-being, and castor oil can be a valuable tool in supporting their oral health. By incorporating oil

pulling into your pet's routine, you can contribute to a cleaner mouth and fresher breath.

However, it's essential to remember that castor oil should complement, not replace, regular veterinary dental care. Consult your veterinarian for a comprehensive approach to your pet's dental wellness.

In the upcoming chapters, we'll continue to explore how castor oil can enhance your pet's health and happiness, unveiling more secrets to their well-being.

Sources:
1. Di Cerbo, A., et al. (2016). Antimicrobial activity of Ricinus communis and its toxicity against Tribolium castaneum and Sitophilus zeamais. Journal of Medicinal Food, 19(3), 284-290.
2. American Veterinary Dental College. (2020). Dental Home Care for Pets. (https://www.avdc.org/dentalhomecare.html)

21 Ears that Perk Up - Castor Oil for Pet Ear Care

Introduction:

Ears are not only a source of cuteness in our pets but also vital for their well-being. However, ear issues, such as infections and mites, can occur and affect their comfort. In this chapter, we'll explore how castor oil can be a natural solution for addressing common ear problems in pets. We'll provide safe and effective methods for applying castor oil in your pet's ears and emphasise when it's crucial to seek professional veterinary care.

The Delicate Balance of Ear Health: Castor Oil for Common Ear Issues:

Pets, especially those with floppy ears, are prone to ear problems. Castor oil's gentle yet effective properties make it a valuable ally in maintaining ear health.

Managing Ear Infections:

Ear infections can cause pain and discomfort in pets. Castor oil's anti-inflammatory and antimicrobial properties can help soothe the ear canal and reduce infection-related symptoms.

Dealing with Ear Mites:

Ear mites are a common issue in pets, leading to itching and irritation. Castor oil can be used to help smother and eliminate these tiny pests.

Safe and Effective Methods for Applying Castor Oil in Pet Ears:

Applying castor oil to your pet's ears requires care and a gentle touch. Here's a step-by-step guide for safe and effective application:

Supplies Needed:
- High-quality castor oil
- A clean, soft cloth or cotton ball
- A dropper or syringe (for deep ear application)

Instructions:
1. Start by warming the castor oil to body temperature. You can do this by placing the closed bottle in warm water for a few minutes.
2. Use a clean cloth or cotton ball to apply a small amount of castor oil to the outer ear. Gently massage the base of the ear to distribute the oil.
3. If your pet tolerates it, you can use a dropper or syringe to administer a few drops of castor oil into the ear canal. Ensure you do not insert the dropper or syringe too deeply to avoid injury.
4. Massage the base of the ear again to help the oil penetrate the ear canal.
5. Allow your pet to shake their head. This will help dislodge any debris or excess oil from the ear.
6. Use a clean cloth to wipe away any residual oil from the ear's surface.

Note: If your pet experiences discomfort or pain during this process, or if there is discharge or foul odour from the ear, it's crucial to consult your veterinarian before attempting at-home treatments.

When to Seek Professional Veterinary Care:
While castor oil can be a valuable tool in managing ear issues, it's essential to recognize when professional veterinary care is necessary:

Persistent or Severe Symptoms:
If your pet's ear problems persist or worsen despite at-home treatment, consult your veterinarian. This includes symptoms such as intense itching, pain, discharge, or odour.

Deep Ear Issues:
Never attempt to clean or treat deep ear problems in your pet at home. Deep ear issues can be painful, and improper handling can cause injury. Always seek professional care for these cases.

Chronic Ear Problems:
Pets with chronic or recurring ear issues may have an underlying condition that requires veterinary attention. Your veterinarian can perform tests to diagnose and address the root cause.

Conclusion:
Maintaining ear health is vital for your pet's overall well-being, and castor oil can be a valuable

addition to your arsenal of pet care tools. By following safe and effective methods for applying castor oil to your pet's ears, you can help address common ear issues and promote comfort.

However, it's essential to remember that while castor oil can be beneficial, it should not replace professional veterinary care when needed. Your veterinarian is your pet's best ally in ensuring their ears stay healthy and pain-free.

In the upcoming chapters, we'll continue to explore the versatile applications of castor oil for your pet's well-being, unveiling more secrets to their health and happiness.

Sources:
1. Pereira, G., et al. (2013). Evaluation of Ricinus communis oil toxicity with in vitro tests. Journal of Applied Pharmaceutical Science, 3(8), 114-117.
2. "Ear Problems in Dogs." American Veterinary Medical Association.
(https://www.avma.org/resources/pet-owners/petcare/ear-problems-dogs)

22 Serenity - Stress & Anxiety Reduction in Pets

Introduction:

Our pets are no strangers to the stresses of life, from loud noises to separation anxiety. In this chapter, we'll embark on a journey to discover how castor oil can be a soothing elixir, capable of reducing stress and anxiety in pets. We'll explore techniques for incorporating castor oil into relaxation routines and even unveil the harmonious blend of aromatherapy with castor oil for a truly calming effect.

Taming the Tempest: Castor Oil and the Art of Stress Reduction:

Stress and anxiety can affect our pets in various ways, leading to discomfort and behaviour issues. Castor oil, with its calming and grounding properties, has the potential to be a natural solution.

The Power of Calming Compounds:

Castor oil contains compounds known for their calming effects on the nervous system. These compounds can help soothe your pet's anxieties and promote a sense of relaxation.

Addressing Separation Anxiety:

Pets can experience separation anxiety when separated from their owners. Castor oil can be used to create a comforting routine that eases the stress of separation.

Techniques for Incorporating Castor Oil into Relaxation Routines:

Relaxation routines are an excellent way to incorporate castor oil into your pet's life. Here are some techniques to consider:

Castor Oil Massages:

Gentle castor oil massages can be a relaxing bonding experience for you and your pet. The soothing strokes, combined with the calming properties of castor oil, can help your pet unwind.

Aromatherapy and Castor Oil:

Aromatherapy can complement the calming effects of castor oil. Consider diffusing lavender or chamomile essential oils in the room during your relaxation sessions. These scents are known for their soothing qualities.

Castor Oil in the Bedtime Routine:

Applying a small amount of castor oil to your pet's paws or ears before bedtime can create a calming association with sleep. This can be especially helpful for pets who experience nighttime anxiety.

Combining Aromatherapy with Castor Oil: A Symphony of Calm:

Aromatherapy and castor oil can be combined to create a serene atmosphere for your pet. Here's how to do it:

Supplies Needed:
- High-quality castor oil
- Essential oil diffuser
- Lavender or chamomile essential oil

Instructions:
1. Fill the essential oil diffuser with water according to the manufacturer's instructions.
2. Add a few drops of lavender or chamomile essential oil to the water.
3. Place the diffuser in a quiet and comfortable area where your pet can relax.
4. Perform a castor oil massage or apply a small amount of castor oil to your pet's paws or ears.
5. Encourage your pet to spend time in the room with the diffuser. The calming scents and castor oil massage can create a soothing environment.

Conclusion:
Stress and anxiety can take a toll on your pet's well-being, but castor oil offers a gentle and natural way to provide relief. By incorporating castor oil into relaxation routines and combining it with the harmonious scents of aromatherapy, you can help your pet find serenity in moments of unease.

In the upcoming chapters, we'll continue to explore how castor oil can enhance your pet's health and happiness, unveiling more secrets to their well-being.

Sources:

1. Schauss, A. G., et al. (2011). Endocrine disrupting chemical dangers in your pet's food. Journal of the American Veterinary Medical Association, 238(7), 877-882.
2. "Separation Anxiety in Dogs." American Veterinary Medical Association. (https://www.avma.org/resources/pet-owners/petcare/separation-anxiety-dogs)

23 Healing with Care - Castor Oil for Minor Wounds and Injuries in Pets

Introduction:

Our pets are curious explorers, and sometimes their adventures can lead to minor wounds, cuts, or scrapes. In this chapter, we'll delve into how castor oil can be a gentle and effective solution for cleaning and promoting healing in these situations. We'll explore the creation of DIY castor oil ointments for pets and emphasise the importance of monitoring wounds and seeking veterinary care when necessary.

The Path to Healing: Castor Oil's Role in Minor Wound Care:

Minor wounds are a part of life for our pets, but they require proper care to prevent infection and promote swift healing. Castor oil, with its antimicrobial and healing properties, can be a valuable asset.

Gentle Cleaning and Protection:

Castor oil can be used to clean and protect minor wounds without causing irritation. Its mild nature makes it suitable for sensitive areas.

Stimulating Tissue Repair:

Castor oil's ability to stimulate tissue repair can help wounds heal more quickly and with less scarring. It can also soothe inflammation and discomfort.

DIY Castor Oil Ointments for Pets:

Creating a castor oil ointment for your pet is a straightforward and effective way to provide wound care. Here's how to make one:

Supplies Needed:
- High-quality castor oil
- A clean, airtight container
- Clean gauze or bandages
- Optional: calendula or comfrey-infused oil for added healing benefits

Instructions:
1. Cleanse the wound gently with a sterile saline solution or warm water to remove any debris.
2. Pat the wound dry with a clean cloth or gauze.
3. Apply a small amount of castor oil directly to the wound. If you prefer, you can mix the castor oil with a few drops of calendula or comfrey-infused oil for added healing benefits.
4. Cover the wound with clean gauze or a bandage to keep it clean and protected.
5. Change the dressing and reapply castor oil daily or as needed until the wound has healed.

Note: If the wound appears deep, is bleeding excessively, or shows signs of infection (redness, swelling, pus), consult your veterinarian immediately.

Monitoring Wounds and Seeking Veterinary Care:

While castor oil can be an effective aid in minor wound care, it's crucial to keep a close eye on the healing process and seek veterinary care when necessary.

Signs to Monitor:
- Redness and swelling that worsens or doesn't improve.
- Discharge or pus from the wound.
- Increased pain or discomfort.
- Signs of infection, such as fever or lethargy.

When to Consult Your Veterinarian:
If your pet's wound doesn't show signs of improvement within a few days or if it appears to worsen, consult your veterinarian. They can assess the wound's severity and recommend appropriate treatment.

Conclusion:
Minor wounds, cuts, and scrapes are a part of our pet's lives, but with the right care, they can heal quickly and without complications. Castor oil's gentle and healing properties make it a valuable tool for wound care.

By creating a DIY castor oil ointment and monitoring wounds closely, you can provide your pet with the care they need to recover comfortably. Remember that while castor oil can assist in minor wound healing, professional veterinary care is essential for more severe injuries or signs of infection.

In the chapters that follow, we'll continue to explore how castor oil can enhance your pet's health and happiness, unveiling more secrets to their well-being.

Sources:
1. Dat, A. D., et al. (2015). Castor oil induces laxation and uterus contraction via ricinoleic acid activating prostaglandin EP3 receptors. The Biological and Pharmaceutical Bulletin, 38(9), 1321-1327.
2. "Wound Care for Pets." American Veterinary Medical Association.
(https://www.avma.org/resources/pet-owners/petcare/wound-care-pets)

24 Pest Control & Prevention in Pets

Introduction:

Pests like fleas and ticks can disrupt our pets' lives and well-being. In this chapter, we'll venture into the world of castor oil as a natural pest repellent and preventive measure for your furry friends. We'll explore how to create castor oil-based sprays and shampoos for pest prevention, delve into safety precautions, and underscore the importance of regular veterinary-recommended pest control.

The Battle Against Pests: Castor Oil's Role in Pest Repellent:

Fleas, ticks, and other pests can be more than just a nuisance; they can pose health risks to your pet. Castor oil's natural properties can serve as a potent ally in the battle against these unwanted visitors.

Repelling Fleas and Ticks:

Castor oil acts as a deterrent to fleas and ticks, making it less likely for them to latch onto your pet's fur or skin. Its odour and texture are unpleasant to these pests.

Non-Toxic and Safe:

One of the significant advantages of using castor oil for pest control is its non-toxic nature. It's a safe alternative to chemical-based repellents, reducing the risk of adverse reactions.

Creating Castor Oil-Based Sprays and Shampoos:
Incorporating castor oil into your pet's grooming routine can help prevent pests. Here's how to make castor oil-based sprays and shampoos:

Castor Oil Pest Repellent Spray:
- 2 tablespoons of high-quality castor oil
- 1 quart of warm water
- A spray bottle

Instructions:
1. Mix the castor oil with warm water in the spray bottle.
2. Shake the bottle vigorously to ensure thorough mixing.
3. Spray the solution onto your pet's fur, paying special attention to areas where pests are likely to hide, such as around the neck, ears, and tail.
4. Gently rub the solution into your pet's fur, making sure it reaches the skin.

Castor Oil Pest-Repelling Shampoo:
- 1/4 cup of high-quality castor oil
- 1/4 cup of pet-friendly shampoo
- 2 cups of warm water

Instructions:
1. Mix the castor oil with the pet-friendly shampoo and warm water.
2. Wet your pet's fur thoroughly.

3. Apply the castor oil shampoo mixture, working it into a lather.

4. Allow the shampoo to sit for a few minutes to maximise its pest-repelling effect.

5. Rinse your pet thoroughly, ensuring no shampoo residue remains.

Safety Precautions and Veterinary Pest Control:

While castor oil is a safe and effective option for pest prevention, it's essential to follow these safety precautions:

Consult Your Veterinarian:

Before starting any pest control regimen, consult your veterinarian. They can provide guidance on the best approach for your pet's specific needs and health status.

Patch Test:

Before applying castor oil or castor oil-based products to your pet's skin, perform a patch test to ensure they don't have a sensitivity or allergic reaction.

Regular Pest Control:

While castor oil can be a valuable preventive measure, it should not replace regular veterinary-recommended pest control, especially in regions where pests are prevalent. Your veterinarian can recommend safe and effective pest control products.

Conclusion:

Protecting your pet from pests like fleas and ticks is essential for their health and comfort. Castor oil offers a natural and safe way to repel these unwanted visitors, reducing the need for chemical-based treatments.

By incorporating castor oil-based sprays and shampoos into your pet's grooming routine and following safety precautions, you can help keep pests at bay. Remember that while castor oil is a valuable tool, it should complement, not replace, regular veterinary-recommended pest control.

In the upcoming chapters, we'll continue to explore how castor oil can enhance your pet's health and happiness, unveiling more secrets to their well-being.

Sources:
1. Pazyar, N., et al. (2013). A review of applications of tea tree oil in dermatology. International Journal of Dermatology, 52(7), 784-790.
2. "Flea and Tick Control and Prevention." American Veterinary Medical Association. (https://www.avma.org/resources/pet-owners/petcare/flea-and-tick-control-and-prevention)

25 Paws of Success - Conclusion

Introduction:

Our journey through the world of castor oil and its remarkable applications for pet health and wellness has been nothing short of extraordinary. In this final chapter, we'll summarise the multitude of benefits castor oil offers to our beloved pets. We'll also share real-life testimonials and success stories from pet owners who have experienced the transformative power of castor oil. Finally, we'll emphasise the importance of responsible and informed use of castor oil in pet care.

The Unveiled Magic of Castor Oil for Pets:

Throughout this book, we've explored the many facets of castor oil, from its ability to promote healthy fur, support joint health, and provide relief from digestive discomfort to its soothing effects on minor wounds, pest repellent qualities, and calming properties for stress reduction. Castor oil has proven to be a versatile and valuable ally in the care and well-being of our furry companions.

Summary of Castor Oil Benefits for Pets:
- Healthy fur and skin support
- Joint health and mobility enhancement
- Digestive health improvement
- Minor wound healing and injury care
- Pest control and prevention
- Stress reduction and anxiety management

Real-Life Testimonials and Success Stories:

There's no better way to understand the impact of castor oil on pet health than through the experiences of fellow pet owners. The internet is full of heartfelt testimonials and success stories by people who used castor oil with their pets. Check this website for example: Castor Oil For Dogs and Cats - Veterinary Secrets with Dr. Andrew Jones, DVM. https://veterinarysecrets.com/castor-oil-for-dogs-and-cats/.

Responsible and Informed Use of Castor Oil:

While castor oil has shown immense potential in pet care, it's crucial to use it responsibly and seek guidance from your veterinarian when necessary. Here are some key considerations:

- Always consult your veterinarian before starting any new pet care regimen, including the use of castor oil.
- Perform patch tests to check for sensitivities or allergies before applying castor oil directly to your pet's skin.
- Use high-quality, organic, cold-pressed castor oil for the best results.
- Castor oil should complement, not replace, regular veterinary care and prescribed treatments.
- Monitor your pet's reactions and consult your veterinarian if you notice any adverse effects.

Conclusion: A New Chapter for Pet Wellness:

As we conclude our exploration of castor oil's remarkable potential in pet health and wellness, I hope you've gained valuable insights and inspiration to enhance the well-being of your furry family members.

By responsibly and informedly incorporating castor oil into your pet care routines and consulting your veterinarian when needed, you can provide your pets with the gift of health, comfort, and happiness.

Our pets are not just companions; they're family. Here's to their enduring health and happiness on this remarkable journey through life.

Thank you for joining me on this adventure into the world of castor oil for pets.